HIV Endurance

HEALTH AND AGING IN THE MARGINS

Series Editor: Alexandra "Xan" C.H. Nowakowski, Florida State University

Health and Aging in the Margins expands the horizons of mainstream and academic understandings of living and aging at the intersection of diverse health experiences and marginalized biographies. Interest in life course perspectives on health and aging has expanded dramatically in recent decades. However, most attention to this topic in extant academic books has focused on more dominant social and cultural groups. This series will build on groundwork laid by these traditions to focus explicitly on the health and aging experiences of marginalized people and groups. These specific topic areas may include but are not limited to:

Racism and People of Color	Kink Practitioners
Stigmatized Conditions	High-Risk Occupations
First-Generation Students	Community and Police Violence
Adoption and Donor Conception	Ethnic Discrimination
Religious and Spiritual Minorities	Asexualities
Working-Class Lives	Invisible Disabilities
Unemployment	Sexism and Feminism
Intimate Partner Violence	Hate Crimes and Survivorship
Food Insecurity	Homelessness and Housing Insecurity
Rare Diseases	Sizeism and Fatphobia
Dementia and Cognitive Impairment	Contested Disorders
Social and Intellectual Differences	Communication Differences
Progressive Diseases	Childfreedom
Trans and Nonbinary Experiences	Infertility and Sterilization
Immigrant and Migrant Families	Gay/Lesbian/Bi/Pan Sexualities
Intersex Lives	Consensual Nonmonogamies
Transgender Studies	Early Mortality

The series centers ethnographic and narrative approaches to explore and understand the health and aging experiences of marginalized populations. Recruitment of authors will focus strongly on amplifying the voices of scholars who themselves have experienced intersectional marginalization and who engage those elements of their personal biography in scholarly activity.

HIV Endurance

Women's Journeys from Diagnosis to Aging

Charlene F. D'Amore

LEXINGTON BOOKS
Lanham • Boulder • New York • London

Published by Lexington Books
An imprint of The Rowman & Littlefield Publishing Group, Inc.
4501 Forbes Boulevard, Suite 200, Lanham, Maryland 20706
www.rowman.com

86-90 Paul Street, London EC2A 4NE

British Library Cataloguing in Publication Information Available

Library of Congress Cataloging-in-Publication Data

Names: D'Amore, Charlene F., 1969- author.
Title: HIV endurance : women's journeys from diagnosis to aging / Charlene F. D'Amore.
Description: Lanham : Lexington Books, [2023] | Series: Health and aging in the margins | Includes bibliographical references.
Identifiers: LCCN 2023027140 (print) | LCCN 2023027141 (ebook) | ISBN 9781666918618 (cloth) | ISBN 9781666918625 (electronic)
Subjects: LCSH: HIV-positive women--United States--Interviews. | HIV-positive women--United States--Social conditions--Interviews. | AIDS (Disease) in women--Social aspects--United States. | Older HIV-positive persons--United States--Interviews. | Older HIV-positive persons--United States--Social conditions--Interviews. | D'Amore, Charlene F., 1969---Health.
Classification: LCC RA643.83 .D36 2023 (print) | LCC RA643.83 (ebook) | DDC 362.19697/920082--dc23/eng/20230719
LC record available at https://lccn.loc.gov/2023027140
LC ebook record available at https://lccn.loc.gov/2023027141

This book is dedicated to the people who fought for the life-saving medications and medical care I benefit from as a woman living with HIV in the United States. My hope is that this level of care proliferates throughout the world so more people living with HIV can live their fullest lives. This book is written in memory of the millions of people who have died from HIV.

Contents

List of Figures and Table

Note to Reader

I wrote this book from a place of privilege which I have partially obtained through my identification as a white, cisgender, college-educated, straight, single, middle-aged woman living in the United States of America. Over my life, I have been fortunate to secure meaningful work that has provided me with a living wage. Additionally, I have health insurance that allows me to obtain quality healthcare and affordable medications. The community where I live helps me to maintain my well-being by providing me with clean, safe, outdoor spaces where I can exercise, engage with my neighbors, purchase healthy foods, and get any necessary services. My life has been free from the experiences of poverty, abuse, violence, inadequate housing and food, discrimination, and marginalization that permeates the lives of many less privileged people. These people who are granted less privileges include some of the women I was honored to briefly meet and interview during my research endeavors. As I wrote this book, I was ever mindful of my sacred duty to accurately convey the words of interview participants and to try to share, to the best of my limited ability, part of their lived experiences. I hope I have not failed in this effort. I appreciate your interest in this subject.

Charlene F. D'Amore, PhD

Preface

My HIV Journey

This preface consists of a sampling from my journal entries from 1998 to 2001, which were the first three years after my HIV diagnosis. By sharing these journal entries, I hope to place the reader into the experience of being diagnosed with HIV. In addition to my case of coping with an HIV diagnosis, you will encounter further examples from the lived experiences of other positive women as you read this book. To protect the identities of all the people in this book, I have assigned them pseudonyms.

MONDAY, JULY 6, 1998

I just got back home after a long holiday weekend. As I unpacked my suitcase, I noticed the light on my answering machine blinking repeatedly. As I listened to my messages, my heartbeat quickened.

> *First message (Thursday, July 2, 1998)*: Hello, this is Dr. Sutherland's office. We are calling to schedule an appointment with Charlene. Please call us back as soon as you get this message.

> *Second message (Friday, July 3, 1998)*: Good afternoon, Charlene. This is Dr. Sutherland's office. Since we still have not heard from you to schedule an appointment, we have scheduled you for a 10:00 a.m. appointment on Monday, July 6 with Dr. Sutherland to go over your blood work results. We look forward to seeing you on Monday at 10 a.m.

> *Third message (Monday, July 6, 1998)*: Hello, Charlene. This is Dr. Sutherland's office. We were disappointed you did not come for your 10:00 a.m. appointment today with Dr. Sutherland. Please call us back as soon as possible so we can schedule you for a follow-up appointment to go over your blood work results.

With a feeling of dread, I called Dr. Sutherland's office, and they scheduled me for an appointment at 11:30 a.m. on Tuesday.

MONDAY, JUNE 29, 1998 (ONE WEEK EARLIER)

Sitting in Dr. Sutherland's exam room, I thought about how tired I was of being sick. When Dr. Sutherland entered the room, I reported I had another bladder infection, my second one in two months.

With a look of sympathy, Dr. Sutherland began to write another prescription for my bladder infection when I interrupted her. I asserted I was tired of being sick and that I had never been this sick before. I reminded her that over the last five months I had two flu infections, several yeast infections, one bacterial infection, and two bladder infections. Every other week I had to come see her for some new infection. To appease me, Dr. Sutherland offered, "Maybe I can request some blood work in addition to giving you a prescription to treat your bladder infection."

I readily agreed to Dr. Sutherland's offer of blood work, and then, I mentioned another concern I had, "Since April, I have had a lump on the base of my head. I think I bumped my head when I fainted during my last flu infection."

Feeling behind my left ear where the lump was located, Dr. Sutherland exclaimed, "That's a swollen lymph node!" As Dr. Sutherland began feeling around my body searching for other swollen lymph nodes, her words reverberated through my body. I had heard the words, "swollen lymph nodes" before when I donated blood a couple of times each year. Those words were part of the screening blood banks administered before they permitted a person to donate. Those words were used to screen out people who may have HIV or AIDS. Blood banks also asked potential donors if they had a recent flu-like infection.

Not finding any other swollen lymph nodes, Dr. Sutherland continued to write my prescription and started to order my blood work when I interrupted her again. "Excuse me Dr. Sutherland, could you also order an HIV test along with my blood work?" Startled, she looked at me questioningly, wondering, I think, why I would need an HIV test considering I was a white, college-educated woman. I elaborated that I had been having unprotected sex with my partner since February, and I just wanted to make sure I didn't have HIV. Nodding, Dr. Sutherland agreed to add an HIV test to my blood work order.

TUESDAY, JULY 7, 1998

When Dr. Sutherland came into the exam room, she uttered the words that altered my life journey, "You are the first person I have ever told this terrible news to. Your HIV test came back positive." I reassured her it was okay and that I had suspected this possibility given my symptoms. Then, Dr. Sutherland said she had called an HIV specialist who requested additional blood work and a chest X-ray. She added her office had scheduled an appointment for me to meet with the HIV specialist on Thursday.

I left Dr. Sutherland's office and went to a nearby radiology office to have my chest X-ray completed. The man conducting the chest X-ray asked me why someone my age, 29 years old, needed a chest X-ray. I informed him I had just been diagnosed with HIV. He asked me how I got it, and I responded I got it through unprotected sex. I saw a look of pity cross his face. I realized then that this was how the rest of my life was going to be, needing to disclose to strangers the most intimate details of my life and then having them judge my choices. I resolved at that moment to not feel victimized or shameful about my new HIV-positive status. After my chest X-ray, I went to a friend's apartment and relayed my devastating news. He was in shock, but he promised he would support me in the months ahead. Back in my apartment, I wrote in my journal through tears before I went to sleep that I hoped to fight this disease with a healthy diet, exercise, and a positive attitude.

WEDNESDAY, JULY 8, 1998

What a long day this has been! I have spent most of my day crying and wallowing in self-pity. I'm thinking about all the things I won't be able to do or have in my life: no wedding, no children, no health, and no longevity. When my partner came to visit tonight, I confessed to him while we sat on my couch that I had tested positive for HIV. At first, he looked shocked and accused me of lying. Then, he sat with his head down, and his eyes closed, repeatedly saying, "I'm going to die." I asked him when his last HIV test was, and he insisted he couldn't remember. I gave him a telephone number to call for a free HIV blood test, but he refused to call, stating he would rather wait to confirm I had HIV. Then, he remarked he would support me but that he wanted to kill himself. I tried to make him feel better by saying there was a chance he did not have HIV.

THURSDAY, JULY 9, 1998

I met with the HIV specialist today. Her name is Susan, and she is a certified nurse practitioner who specializes in caring for people living with HIV. Susan interviewed me and concluded I had been infected with HIV from my current sexual partner. I argued that I had spoken to my partner before we had sex, and he had assured me that he had tested negative for HIV. With disbelief, I asked, "You don't think someone would lie about testing negative for HIV?" Susan responded, "Has he lied to you about anything else?" Slowly, I realized he had lied to me about other things over the last couple of months. Susan then emphasized there could be no other possibility since I had donated blood a month before I met my partner in February, and my flu-like infections had been in March and April.

I asked Susan why I had two flu-like infections, and she suggested I was probably infected twice. Looking back on my calendar, I determined I had oral sex with my partner on the same day I had gone to the dentist for a routine cleaning. The following day, I remember having a burning sensation on the roof of my mouth, and five days later, I had my first flu-like symptoms. The second infection was from vaginal intercourse after I had been treated for genital warts. The scab from having my warts frozen had come off during intercourse. Susan explained the virus had entered through that opening, causing my second flu-like infection in April. Then, Susan gave me some reading material about the virus and scheduled me to return on Thursday, July 16 to discuss my blood work results. She also urged me to encourage my partner to get tested.

THURSDAY, JULY 16, 1998

I have been reading a lot about HIV and how it affects people. I learned the virus reproduces new viruses at a rate of 10 billion a day! I really do not want to start taking HIV drugs, but at this rate of viral production, I might not have a choice. I hope my numbers aren't too high, but I did have two infections of HIV. Over the past couple of days, I have been looking for more books about HIV. I went to several bookstores, but they didn't have any books about living with HIV. I then went to the library and found only one book about people living with HIV. However, I was very fortunate to discover a cassette tape with some readings from a book entitled *From a Burning House: The AIDS Project Los Angeles Writers Workshop Collection*. I have listened to the tape every night and cried because it contains the words of gay men who have lived and died of AIDS in Los Angeles.

In the exam room with Susan, she shared my blood test results. My CD4 count was 240! The normal range is 800 to 1200. My viral load was 340,000! Anything over 10,000 is considered high risk. Susan recommended I begin taking the antiretroviral medications immediately. She explained the goal was to keep the viral count as low as possible to slow the reproduction of the virus. I complained I didn't want to commit to taking pills every day, and I asked if there was any alternative. Susan repeated it was better not to wait, and there was no other alternative to the antiretroviral medications. I decided to listen to her advice, and she ordered several prescriptions for me.

When I informed my sexual partner about my test results, he countered that he had gone for an HIV test, and his test had come back negative. I asked him to show me his test results, but he refused to produce any papers. I then challenged that I wanted to go with him for a free state health department test, but he refused to go. Because of his refusal, I decided to contact my previous sexual partners and the blood bank where I had donated in January to inform them of my positive status. When I called my previous sexual partners, they were in shock and admonished me for having unprotected sex. They blamed me and scolded me that I should have known better. Also, they all assured me they had recent negative HIV test results. Then, they offered their support to me. After these disclosures, I confronted my current sexual partner again and accused him of lying about his test results, but he continued to be in a deep, deep, denial.

TUESDAY, AUGUST 11, 1998

I have now focused my time and energy on learning how to live with HIV. Every day, I read a lot, especially about other people who are living with HIV. Susan gave me several *POZ* magazines. I have read every article in them. I really appreciate seeing and reading about other people who are living with HIV. Reading the *POZ* magazines gives me hope I too can live a normal, productive life with HIV. I have also called various hotlines and helplines for advice and comfort. The organization Project Inform has been the most helpful. I have called Project Inform several times to ask questions about how to take my antiretroviral medications and about the side effects of each drug. The men who I have spoken to have given me their honest, first-hand experiences with these medications and how to manage the daily dose of pills. They have also helped me by suggesting proactive steps I can take to live a healthy life.

Another especially helpful hotline has been HIV Nightline. I call them when I am at my most desperate and depressed times, which is always in the middle of the night when I can't sleep because I am crying so much. The men at HIV Nightline have talked me through my crying bouts and helped me calm down. They help me to realize an HIV diagnosis is not a death sentence anymore because of the antiretroviral medications now available.

Susan also gave me the phone number of a trainer who works with people who are living with HIV. He gave me information about nutrition and strength training exercises. I have started taking my antiretroviral medications. My initial side effects were nausea, vomiting, and fatigue. Now, my side effects have lessened. I have also started working again.

FRIDAY, NOVEMBER 13, 1998

My viral load has dropped from 340,000 to 31,000, and now to 7,000! My exercising and diet have improved greatly also. I'm back to full-time work, and my energy and stamina have returned. My partner and I are still together, but we don't talk about HIV because it causes a big argument. I'm not ready yet to break up with him because I don't want to be alone. Also, I am not ready yet to date other people and disclose my HIV-positive status to them. I was able to order a copy of the book *From a Burning House: The AIDS Project Los Angeles Writers Workshop Collection*. I have read it twice already. The essays are teaching me how to live and die with HIV. I still call Project Inform and HIV Nightline occasionally for advice and to speak to other people who are living with HIV. I'm also still reading *POZ* magazines and any other information I can find about HIV and AIDS.

FRIDAY, FEBRUARY 19, 1999

Today, I met with my partner's best friend, and I divulged I was HIV-positive. Shocked by my news, he promised he would make sure my partner went and got tested. So far, my main support people have been my friend, who was the first person I disclosed to, and Susan.

SATURDAY, MARCH 6, 1999

I learned today my partner is HIV-positive also. I went to the state health department with him to get the results. His counts were 204 for CD4 cells and 35,000 for viral load. I offered to introduce him to my HIV specialist, but he refused to go. We are drifting further apart, and I realize I'm going to have to move away to separate from him.

FRIDAY, APRIL 9, 1999

Susan asked me to present with her on the topic of women living with HIV. She is going to speak to some other medical staff to increase their awareness of HIV's effects on women. At first, I was adamant that I didn't want to talk to anyone about HIV. However, Susan argued people needed to see and hear from me because I don't fit people's preconceived notions about HIV-positive women. After some consideration and with Susan's encouragement, I agreed to speak publicly because I perceived I was able to speak about living with HIV, and other women might not be comfortable disclosing in public. I also realized how privileged I was to be able to take antiretroviral medications and that the medications worked for me. I kept telling myself, "I need to do more than just financially support some AIDS Service Organizations. I need to speak to help prevent additional HIV infections."

SATURDAY, MAY 15, 1999

This past week, I informed my older sister and brother-in-law that I was HIV-positive when I spoke to them over the telephone. I also told my older brother and his wife while we sat in their car. Additionally, I divulged my positive status to my parents today while standing in their kitchen. All my family members were in shock, but they also are being supportive. I gave them brochures with information about people living with HIV and some phone numbers to call for information.

SATURDAY, JUNE 5, 1999

Today, I spoke for the second time to a group of people about living with HIV as a woman. I spoke to about 100 healthcare providers and pharmacists with Susan, my HIV specialist. Another woman joined us. She has lived with HIV for the past ten years! Her name was Christine. Afterward, we went out to eat and became fast friends. Christine related how she became infected with HIV, and I shared how I became infected. Then, Christine told me about her work and her family, and I spoke about my work and family. Christine mentioned she was a member of a group called Women Organized to Respond to Life-Threatening Diseases (WORLD), and she gave me a couple of their newsletters to read. This is the first group I have heard about for women living with HIV. It was nice to read about other women and about their advocacy work. I really enjoyed meeting Christine. Her life experiences living with HIV for over ten years have inspired me to persevere.

THURSDAY, SEPTEMBER 16, 1999

I spoke to another sixty nurses and counselors today about being a newly diagnosed woman living with HIV. Susan spoke first. Then, I spoke about my experiences over the past year. Then, Christine spoke about her experiences during the early years of the AIDS epidemic, which were in stark contrast to my experiences. She encountered several incidences of stigma when medical providers learned she was HIV-positive. Christine also refused to take the early antiretroviral medications because she feared the medications' side effects, but now, she is on antiretroviral therapy. Over her many years of living with HIV, Christine has always worked full-time, and she got married several years ago. Speaking to Christine gives me hope for my future. I broke up with my partner over the summer. I have also moved to another state and started a new job. Now, I am struggling trying to negotiate dating as a woman living with HIV.

TUESDAY, OCTOBER 12, 1999

Over the weekend, I attended the National Conference on Women and HIV in Los Angeles. Over 1,000 women were there! I got to hear a lot of speakers and other women sharing their experiences living with HIV.

THURSDAY, JANUARY 6, 2000

During the holiday season, I revealed to my two best friends from college that I was HIV-positive. They were both supportive. In December, I also attended my first HIV retreat, where I met other people living with HIV. I participated in some support group discussions at the retreat. This retreat caused a lot of emotional pain to come to the surface because I was struggling with how to incorporate HIV into my identity and my religious beliefs. I was also trying to start the process of forgiving my ex-partner and myself.

TUESDAY, JANUARY 25, 2000

Today, I met with my new infectious disease doctor. He is very knowledgeable about HIV. However, he wants me to increase my protease inhibitors to try to lower my viral load more. My last blood work indicated my viral load was around 80, and my CD4 count was 450. I protested that I was not going to take more of my protease inhibitors. He wants me to reach an undetectable level, but I don't want to increase my protease inhibitors. I agreed to get another series of blood tests to see what my new counts are. I wish I had more courage to speak about sexually transmitted infections and HIV prevention, so I could encourage other women to get tested. I know my experiences would help other women if only I can gather the courage to share my story more.

MONDAY, MAY 1, 2000

Over the weekend, I was presenting again with Susan and Christine. We were speaking to a group of graduate nursing students. I was a little apprehensive because I recognized one of the students in the group. I'm not sure if the student recognized me. I was also extra emotional and frustrated about feeling as if I am living two different lives and personas. I have my life and self before I became HIV-positive and now my life and self as a woman living with HIV. I don't know how to bring these two different worlds together. I'm still so scared of people finding out I am living with HIV. I still feel ashamed and blame myself for becoming HIV-positive.

TUESDAY, JUNE 13, 2000

I spoke to a foundation today by myself. The foundation is raising money for legal services and HIV prevention. I emphasized the importance of legal assistance for people living with HIV. I also reported the limited availability of these services for people in the area. After speaking to the members of the foundation's board of directors, I met a friend for lunch. When he asked me why I was in the area, I related I was speaking about HIV prevention. He inquired how I got interested in that topic, and I revealed I was living with HIV. My friend was surprised to learn this, but he was supportive.

MONDAY, JULY 17, 2000

I divulged to my younger sister today that I was HIV-positive. I told her in my parents' living room with my older sister nearby. My younger sister asked several questions and promised she would be supportive of me. Over the weekend, I attended my second HIV retreat. I ascertained I have a lot of work to do around the topics of religion, spirituality, and HIV. I need to find peace with these topics, resolve my guilt and shame around living with HIV, and forgive myself and my ex-partner.

WEDNESDAY, AUGUST 16, 2000

Last night, I spoke to a group of nurse practitioners, and I spoke to a group of business executives this morning. Both presentations went well. I am feeling more confident speaking in front of people about my experiences as a newly diagnosed woman living with HIV.

SUNDAY, AUGUST 20, 2000

Over the weekend, I informed my younger brother that I was HIV-positive. Now, everyone in my immediate family knows. My brother asked questions and assured me of his support. I am so blessed to have the support of my family and friends. I know many people living with HIV are not as fortunate as I am to have the love and support of others.

SUNDAY, MARCH 4, 2001

HIV—Those three letters carry so much weight and meaning. Thank God for the medicines I have the privilege to take. Many people living with HIV do not have the opportunity to take these life-saving drugs. I feel guilty that I have the ability and means to take the antiretrovirals and that they work for me. I also ask myself why I have the privilege of still living after three years of having HIV. I know if I didn't have access to and the ability to take the antiretroviral medications, I would be dead.

WEDNESDAY, MARCH 14, 2001

Today, I presented on my own to about fifty college students, mostly women. I started to cry while I was driving home after my presentation because I wondered if my talk made any difference and if the women would change their behaviors and practice safer sex after hearing about my experiences.

SUNDAY, APRIL 1, 2001

This weekend, I attended my third weekend retreat for people living with HIV. I started crying right after I arrived. I am tired of crying, and I wonder how many more stages of grief I need to go through before I have resolved my feelings of anger, disappointment, and sadness. I wish I could speed up this process. It is so painful to go through these emotions and memories.

WEDNESDAY, JUNE 13, 2001

Millions of people are dying of AIDS in Africa. Young girls and babies are being raped and sodomized because tribal leaders tell men it's a way to rid themselves of the virus. I need to do more to educate people about HIV and to help end this pandemic. I am in the process of moving again, and I am going to begin to prepare myself to become more of a leader in HIV prevention and education. First, I need to work on my spiritual life and continue to work on forgiving myself and my ex-partner. I also need to unify my pre-HIV self with my current HIV self. Then, I need to increase my leadership skills.

SINCE JUNE 2001

From 2001 to 2010, I worked on my spiritual development and on unifying my pre-HIV identity with my current HIV identity. I continued to occasionally speak publicly about living with HIV, especially to college students. I returned to getting my HIV care from Susan, and I changed to a different antiretroviral therapy, which brought my viral load to undetectable. Additionally, I met a couple of times each year with Christine for dinner, a walk, and to renew our friendship. Speaking to Christine helped me to set goals and to stay inspired. Christine connected me with a spiritual development workshop that I attended multiple times each year for intense spiritual work. Because

I wanted to focus on myself, my work, and my life, I minimized dating and concentrated on developing myself and my inner world.

In 2011, I started working on my PhD in administration and leadership studies. When it came time to write my dissertation, I decided I wanted to research women's experiences with HIV disclosure. I had disclosed publicly before I told my family because I feared my family's reactions, and I needed my family's support and love. I recognized how blessed I was to have loving and supportive friends and family who bolstered me along my HIV journey. For me, speaking publicly was a way I could contribute a little to reduce the spread of HIV. I wondered how my disclosure experiences were different from other women who were living with HIV. I set out to interview women about their disclosure experiences. The women I spoke to not only shared their disclosure experiences, they also revealed how they are living and aging with HIV.

Acknowledgements

My first acknowledgement is to the seventeen women participants who volunteered their time to share their lived experiences with me. I am grateful for their willingness to participate in my interviews and to share a little of their lives with HIV. Their words may act as beacons of hope for other women living and aging with HIV.

Next, I wish to acknowledge the support and encouragement I have received from my colleagues in a monthly writers' support group. By participating in a support group, I have benefitted from the wise counsel of others and been inspired by their accomplishments.

Because so much of this book is based on the data and writing I completed while working on my dissertation, I want to acknowledge the support and guidance I received from my dissertation chairwoman and my dissertation committee. Through many revisions, my dissertation was improved. I appreciate the guidance my committee and chairwoman gave me throughout my dissertation writing process.

Now, I would like to express my appreciation for the reviewers who read early drafts of this book and offered me invaluable critiques. This appreciation also includes the wonderful support and encouragement I received from the staff of Lexington Books and Rowman & Littlefield. Your insights and suggestions have improved the final copy of this book and helped me to be a better writer. Thank you for the opportunity to work with you on this project.

Finally, I wish to acknowledge the love and support I have received from my family and friends who have prayed for my success and encouraged me to pursue my dreams and life purpose. I have drawn on their love and support to sustain my journey with HIV and to build my HIV endurance.

Introduction

Hearing you have tested positive for HIV is devastating. A person immediately begins to contemplate who to tell and how to tell others this crushing news. The goal of this book is to serve as a guide for women living with HIV as they navigate disclosing their HIV-positive status to others, encountering situations involving HIV stigma, incorporating HIV into their identity, and aging with HIV. The contents of this book may also inform other readers who are health and social service providers, fellow social science researchers, and other people who support women who are living with HIV. In the preface, I describe the start of my HIV journey as a white, college-educated, cisgender, straight, single woman. In the remainder of the book, I draw from my qualitative research involving seventeen women who are also living with HIV to provide guidance for other positive women and their care providers. I interviewed these women from 2015 to 2016, and they mainly live in and around the cities of Baltimore, Maryland; Philadelphia and Pittsburgh, Pennsylvania; Washington, D.C., and Wilmington, Delaware. As I declared in the preface, all the people named in this book have been given pseudonyms to protect their identities.

This book is divided into four main sections. The first section focuses on the results from my disclosure research. In the first chapter, I summarize the disclosure experiences of the participants from my qualitative research. I then offer a review of additional disclosure research and propose a model of HIV disclosure based on my research findings. After that, I explore the differences between private sphere disclosures, transitional disclosures, and public sphere disclosures. I then outline some of the rationale and results of disclosure and nondisclosure. The first section ends with disclosure advice offered from the lived experiences of my interviewees to other women who are living with HIV.

The second section focuses on the experiences of stigma and strategies to challenge the societal stigma associated with HIV. First, the women I interviewed share some of their experiences of HIV stigma. Then, I offer a summary of research on the causes, factors, and effects of HIV stigma. After that, I focus on strategies to challenge HIV stigma.

In the third section, an analysis of how HIV affects a woman's identity and how she copes with living with HIV is presented. This section opens with the voices of the women I interviewed who share how HIV has affected their lives and how they cope with living with HIV every day. Then, I present research about how living with a chronic illness affects a person's identity and how a diagnosis of HIV acts as an ambiguous loss and a traumatic event in a person's life. Using research on how people try to preserve themselves after a traumatic event, I apply these efforts to women living with HIV. I then share an autoethnographic description of my efforts to incorporate HIV into my identity while preserving myself.

The fourth section examines the experience of aging with HIV. This section is divided into three parts. The first part outlines the personal concerns of some interview participants as they live with HIV in their 50s and 60s. The second part summarizes some research findings on aging with HIV. The third part offers some suggestions for individuals, organizations, and society to sustain HIV endurance as people age with HIV.

At the end of each section, I offer a personal connection and a list of four key takeaways to summarize the main content of each section. At the end of the book, the conclusion connects the information shared in this book with the *National HIV/AIDS Strategy for the United States 2022–2025* [*Strategy*] to offer additional ways to build and sustain HIV endurance. In the appendices, there is a list of additional resources, a glossary of terminology associated with the HIV epidemic, and a summary of the spiritual principles that have sustained me during my HIV journey.

SECTION I

HIV Disclosure

Chapter 1

Other Women's HIV Journeys

From August 2015 to August 2016, I interviewed seventeen women to learn about their HIV disclosure experiences and their life journeys with HIV. All the women volunteered to speak to me and signed informed consent forms, which had been approved by my university's Institutional Review Board as part of my dissertation research. The women mostly lived in and around the cities of Baltimore, Maryland; Philadelphia and Pittsburgh, Pennsylvania; Washington, D.C.; and Wilmington, Delaware. Fourteen of the women identified as African Americans; two women identified as white; and one described herself as Hispanic. Seven of the women were diagnosed before 1997, which was the year antiretroviral therapy became the standard of HIV care in the United States (amfAR, 2022).

Twelve of the women were over 50 years of age, and the oldest woman was 68. Describing their marital status, nine women identified as single; five women answered they were married; and three women revealed they were widowed. Five of the women are public speakers and advocates for HIV prevention. This chapter summarizes the experiences of some of these women when they received their HIV diagnosis and their subsequent disclosure events. Because the experience of HIV diagnosis and disclosure varied over time due to society's views of HIV, I am dividing participants according to the decade of their HIV diagnosis and offering some historical context for each period.

THE 1980S

In the United States, AIDS was first identified in a woman in August 1981, shortly after it was identified as an unusual cancer in young, gay men in San Francisco and New York City, in June 1981 (Farmer et al., 2011). By 1983, the Centers for Disease Control and Prevention (CDC) published a report on women and AIDS (Farmer et al., 2011). In 1987, the first antiretroviral medication, AZT, began to be used to treat people who were living with HIV (amfAR, 2022). According to Farmer et al. (2011), in 1988, African American women's incidence of AIDS was 11 times higher than white women, and the death rate from HIV was nine times higher for African American women than for white women. Two of my research participants received their HIV diagnoses in the 1980s as summarized next.

Irene

After learning her husband was diagnosed with AIDS in 1985, Irene got tested and found out she was also HIV-positive. About a month later, Irene shared her secret with her mother, who had always been understanding. Irene's mother was supportive of Irene and her husband after hearing the devastating news. Additionally, Irene described the difficulty of keeping HIV secret from her family and friends because, although she had always been very honest and open, people didn't talk about AIDS during the 1980s. Feeling like a "walking time bomb," Irene explained, "There was no medication at first, and then, there was one medication that came out, which was AZT. If that medication didn't work, it's like, sorry."

Irene chose not to share her HIV-positive status with anyone else after disclosing it to her mother. She related, "I was very reserved initially, aside from telling my mother, and then, it was something that I held inside of me for a while. It was just hard holding that in and not being able to talk about it." So, one day, in 1987, Irene disclosed in a news article; however, her workplace found out and immediately fired her after eight and a half years of faithful service. Additionally, Irene's church congregation soon discovered she was HIV-positive. At first, the church leaders promised they would support her. However, the leaders then asked Irene to discontinue her work with the children in the church's nursery because they feared she would transmit the virus to the children. Soon after, Irene was asked by the church leaders to find a new church for herself and her family.

After her first husband died, Irene, who is white, married another man who was also living with HIV. Determined to help educate people, especially students, about HIV prevention, Irene completed training in HIV prevention. Since 1999, Irene and her husband have spoken about HIV prevention in schools. During her interview, Irene revealed, "When I speak publicly, it's very therapeutic; it's very hard; I always cry in the end as I'm sharing the personal, emotional side, but they know it's real."

Nevaeh

As an African American teenager in 1989, Nevaeh discovered she was living with HIV. Two days after finding out, Nevaeh contacted a minister friend seeking guidance and consolation. During our interview, Nevaeh said, "I was close to her, and I needed to share with someone 'cause I didn't know what to do. She was worried about me, but she reacted fine. She was definitely a support for me. She supported me before my mother did. I told my mother the day I found out. She didn't react well. She told me not to tell nobody, and she didn't wanna talk about it."

Nevaeh said that her minister friend helped her to really rely on her faith. Over time, Nevaeh disclosed to additional family members and friends. She declared, "I always have disclosed because it's part of—the HIV is part of who I am and so I feel like if you're gonna accept me, then you have to accept all of me." When asked how she disclosed her status to her family and friends, Nevaeh replied, "I just—I told 'em—I just told 'em, and I left it up to them how they were gonna react to it." Nevaeh shared the reactions of her family and friends as, "Mostly positive. I've had some rejection, but then, I figure they really weren't my friends; and they really didn't love me anyway if they rejected me, so."

THE 1990S

In the United States, AIDS was perceived as a disease mostly affecting gay men, and according to Farmer et al. (2011), women were not thought of as vulnerable, as portrayed in the 1990 book *The Myth of Heterosexual AIDS*. African American women were especially marginalized because of racism, gender inequality, and poverty, which put them at greater risk of contracting HIV, while having less access to medical treatment (Farmer et al., 2011). As a result, by 1991, African Americans accounted for 30% of all reported AIDS cases, even though they represented only 12% of the population of the United States (Farmer et al., 2011). Additionally, in 1991, AIDS had become the leading cause of death among young urban women, who were mostly infected with HIV through heterosexual intercourse (Farmer et al., 2011). After intense lobbying, the CDC changed the definition of AIDS to include the most common reproductive tract infections that women experienced, which resulted in a tripling of the number of women diagnosed with AIDS in 1992 (Farmer et al., 2011). By 1993, the number of women reported to be living with AIDS had risen to 16,000 according to Farmer et al. (2011).

Furthermore, by 1992, the number of new HIV transmissions was relatively constant at around 40,000 transmissions annually according to amfAR (2022). However, due to the increased use of protease inhibitors and three drug antiretroviral therapies, which were first introduced at the XI International Conference on AIDS in 1996, people were living longer with HIV, and the number of people dying of AIDS was greatly reduced in the United States (Feldman & Miller, 1998). In 1998, however, African American leaders began to express their concerns about the devastation AIDS was inflicting on their communities because of the lack of access to quality health-care for African Americans living with HIV (amfAR, 2022). By 1999, women accounted for 23% of all AIDS cases in the United States, and roughly one-third of all new HIV transmissions were occurring in women, especially in women younger than age 30 (amfAR, 2022).

Out of the seventeen women I interviewed, seven of them had received their HIV diagnosis in the 1990s. I will now share the diagnosis and disclosure experiences of some of these participants.

Laila

After giving birth to her daughter in 1992, Laila, who is African American, learned she was living with HIV. An active user of drugs, Laila denied her positive status and continued to use drugs, declaring:

> At that time, I was like, I really thought of it as a death sentence; and the way that I was told [when I went to pick my daughter up at the hospital] was very, very disturbing. I guess, and back then, yeah, twenty-four years ago, it wasn't [African Americans weren't] very educated on it and when you heard it, you thought, automatically, death. And for me, I was like, 'Oh well, I'm dying—I'ma die.' So, I had the mindset that 'Hey, I'ma take everybody I could take with me, and I'ma smoke awhile I'm going.' and that was my mindset.

It wasn't until three or four years after finding out she was HIV-positive that Laila finally disclosed her status as she recalled:

> Yeah, I had kids at home. I had two already, a girl—my oldest son and my oldest daughter. The Child and Family man came to my door. Yeah, so from that point, I can honestly say that's where my help started; and I ended up going, talking to the judge and everything, and I told them that I needed help because I was on crack cocaine; and I needed help, and I wanted to go in treatment 'cause I wanted to stop. And they sent me to detox and that is where I told a therapist that I was HIV-positive.

Kendra

After years of drug addiction, Kendra, an African American woman, discovered she was living with HIV in 1993. Crying and very upset by the devastating news, Kendra went home and informed her partner that she had tested positive for HIV. His initial shock soon turned to support. Still "scared to death," Kendra turned to a friend, "Because I was upset, and they could tell. I just came out and told 'em. It was no preparation because it was really not anticipated that I was gonna be upset at that moment. I just broke down at that moment." Over the next ten years, Kendra eventually told one of her sisters and one of her brothers, but she was still reluctant to share much of her personal life with others.

Tamara

Finding out she was living with HIV after being admitted to the hospital, Tamara immediately disclosed it to her eldest sister. Recounting her reason for immediately disclosing, Tamara recalled:

> We already had a sister that was living with an AIDS diagnosis, and it was not something new in my family. [My eldest sister,] she took it very well. She wanted to make sure I was okay and was real supportive; and at that time, she told me just to come home and stay with her 'til I got on my feet, which I did. In my family, there has been no negative response to me disclosing my status whatsoever. The only thing that they wanted to make sure of is, like, give me more information what it is because back in 1996 we were just coming into, especially the African American community, of like, what is this? Even though we had a sister and we had a cousin who passed away, but like what is this virus? How do you live with this virus, and how's it transmitted—and things like that were their concerns—and as I educated myself, I educated them as well.

Still in college and actively dating, Tamara revealed her disclosure strategy with her past sexual partners:

> I've had several partners. My experience with past partners has always been successful because I don't talk about my status when I'm dating someone and it's just like a date, a dinner or something. I want them to find out who I am first, right? And if that relationship moves on to be something bigger, and we want to take it to another level, such as a sexual encounter, then I will set the thing for me to disclose to them in a safe environment, which is my home or in my doctor's office. That way if it doesn't go well, I'm not leaving, and they have to leave; and I'm still supported in my home or in my doctor's office or with someone else that I brought along as I disclosed; but fortunately, I have never had a bad experience because I've educated myself, and I have been able

> to articulate to people who I have dated who are not positive about transmission, what the virus is actually is—and I articulate how well I was doing. I brought my CD4 count and my viral load, and after all that kind of information, so it's went well in the past. I'm currently married to a wonderful, wonderful man who's negative.

Destiny

A self-described workaholic, Destiny talks and moves quickly. After being hospitalized with pneumonia in 1998, Destiny learned she had almost died of AIDS. Because she had been celibate for years, Destiny didn't believe the doctor when he informed her that she had AIDS. She left the hospital and went home. Destiny immediately told her mother and her children who were ages 15 and 20. She then called her friends and divulged to them because:

> I was in shock and so were they. I was like, 'Can you believe that this is what they told me?' That's where I was at—'Can you believe this is what they told me?' And they were like, 'Oh my God, are you serious?' And I was like, 'Yes, I'm serious.' And I was upset; I cried; I threw the papers on the floor; I didn't want none of that stuff; I told them they were wrong, and I said, 'I'm going home, and I'm gonna tell my family.' And that's what I did. When they released me from the hospital, I said, 'I have something I have to tell you.' And my daughter said, 'Is it bad mom?' She's the oldest. And I said, 'Yes, it is.' And she started getting scared, and her and my son sat down, and my mom, and I told 'em, and they start crying.

After disclosing to her family and friends, Destiny, who is African American, regained her health and stamina. Her family and friends were very supportive. They prepared food and took care of her. After recovering from her pneumonia, Destiny was able to return to her busy daily work schedule and was able to reduce her viral load to undetectable by adhering to her antiretroviral medications.

THE 2000S

The Global Fund to Fight AIDS, Tuberculosis, and Malaria was established in 2002, and the first rapid HIV-1 antibody test was approved (amfAR, 2022). Furthermore, in 2003, President George W. Bush started PEPFAR, which was a five-year, $15 billion initiative to fight HIV in Africa and the Caribbean (amfAR, 2022). By 2005, the CDC reported that more than one million Americans were living with HIV, and in 2006, African Americans accounted for more than half of the new HIV transmissions in the United

States (amfAR, 2022). In 2009, the United States House of Representatives removed the 20-year ban on federal funding for syringe exchange programs and the ban from 1987 that restricted travel to the United States by visitors or immigrants who have HIV (amfAR, 2022). Additionally, the White House set goals to reduce HIV transmissions, to increase access to care, and to reduce health disparities through a national HIV strategy in 2010 (amfAR, 2022).

While much progress was made fighting the AIDS epidemic from 1981 to 2010, blaming the victim is a recurrent theme in the AIDS epidemic, as with other epidemics such as tuberculosis (Farmer et al., 2011). In the United States, HIV prevention messages have always emphasized personal agency. However, it is unfair to use personal agency as a basis of assigning blame when most women living with HIV are poor with limited resources. Lacking the opportunity to exert agency in their lives, these women have been blamed, silenced, and unheard, even when they have tried to speak and organize (Farmer et al., 2011). According to Berger (2004), popular notions about AIDS laid the burden and blame on women, especially sex workers, who were not considered among the worthy victims of AIDS, which included children, hemophiliacs, and monogamous heterosexual women who acquired the virus from a gay or bisexual husband. Five of the seventeen women who I interviewed were diagnosed with HIV during the 2000s, and some of their diagnosis and disclosure experiences are summarized next.

Ava

An outgoing and friendly African American woman, Ava enjoys connecting with and helping other people. Ava found out she was living with HIV in 2000. Believing she had received the virus from her ex-husband, Ava felt a responsibility to inform her current sexual partner, who was incarcerated. Ava shared her first disclosure experiences:

> I had been dating him since 1999. I went up to the jail, and I told him two days after I found out. I thought that was the safest place for me to come out with it—I said, 'Well, he's locked up, so he can't kill me.' Come to find out this person had been positive since '91, but they didn't believe it during that time. It went bad for me and him because first of all, he never believed it when he got tested way back then—like, 'I'm not gay; I'm not messin' with men, so no, I can't have that virus.'—'cause during those years, like '91 or whatever, they still considered it a gay man's disease. So, he didn't believe the test, and then to find out that he gave it to me with his non-belief when he could a done something about it was really hard; and for me to know that we waited a year and six months even before having sex. For me that being a monogamous relationship with this person and for me to contract the disease; I was shocked; I was hurt; I was confused. I was on a self-destructive pattern of drugs and alcohol. That

> first [disclosure] experience prepared me that trying to kill myself was not the right thing to do. Basically, after I told him, I let my [teenage] daughter know, because we had a close, loving relationship, and I thought that she should know. I felt a little bit more comfortable knowing that she knew.

Josie

After becoming a widow, Josie, who is African American, started dating again in her late fifties. She was surprised when she tested positive for HIV in 2006. After finding out, Josie went home and called her best friend on the telephone. "Guess what? I'm HIV-positive. I walked in the clinic, asked to be tested, got tested, and drove myself home."

Josie went on to describe how she kept a list of who she disclosed to over the next couple of months:

> There were a few people I hesitated to tell 'cause I didn't want to have to go through no crap with them, and I knew they were the ones that would come up with the crap; but I told my best friend and a couple other close friends. I told my brother, that I'm very close to. I didn't tell my sister 'cause I'm not close to her. So yeah, I was selective at first, and I actually kept a list of who I told. I had an address book and on the back page I was writing names—just names—and when I got to, the page was full, I was like, 'Why are you writing names? You probably told more people than you haven't told.' So, I stopped then. Then, it was just I was out there, and I was speaking six months after diagnosis.

Michelle

After 25 years of drug use, Michelle discovered she was living with HIV in 2007. She immediately called her family members and asked them to gather at her mother's house. Michelle, who is African American, reported to them about her HIV diagnosis because she was in shock and was hoping for their support. Unfortunately, her family was not very supportive, because, although she had stopped using drugs in 2000 and was in a treatment program, her family still blamed her positive status on her lifestyle. During her interview, Michelle reported:

> After the doctor told me I was positive, I asked her, 'Okay, what do I do first?' And she said, 'I recommend that you tell your family.' And that's what I did. I didn't remember how I got to my mother's house, and I told everybody—my mom was there; my father was there; the siblings. They were sorry for me. But now that they know I have it, they don't call and check on me. It hurts me, but they just don't. I guess they think, 'Well, I'm sorry she's got it.' But they don't call and keep up with me.

THE 2010S

During the 2010s, there was more hope in finding a cure for HIV or at least getting more people to an undetectable viral load. In 2011, the CDC announced that only 30% of the people living with HIV in the United States were controlling their viral load, while around 60% of people living with HIV were not receiving medical care (amfAR, 2022). In 2012, the United States Department of Health and Human Services recommended all adults and adolescents living with HIV receive antiretroviral treatments because a low viral load greatly reduces the transmission rate of HIV (amfAR,2022). Also, the Food and Drug Administration (FDA) approved the first at-home HIV test and the use of pre-exposure prophylaxis for HIV negative adults in 2012 (amfAR, 2022). Additionally, because the travel ban was lifted against people living with HIV, the International AIDS Conference held the first United States conference since 1990 in Washington, DC in 2012 (amfAR, 2022).

In 2014, major parts of the Patient Protection and Affordable Care Act (2010)—specifically the provision that insurance companies could not discriminate against people who have pre-existing conditions such as HIV—went into effect (amfAR, 2022). Still in 2017, African Americans, who comprise 13% of the United States' population, accounted for 43% of new HIV diagnoses (amfAR, 2022).

Out of the seventeen interviews I conducted in 2015 to 2016, three women were diagnosed with HIV in the 2010s, and two of these women's experiences are summarized next.

Hailey

Shocked and angry, Hailey expounded on how she discovered she was HIV-positive at a methadone clinic in 2011:

> Well, when they first told me, 'cause I found out 'cause I was on the methadone program, and they tested my blood; and it came back abnormal, so then they told me; they disclosed I had to go to the health clinic, that I was HIV-positive, and for like fifteen years, I was a intravenous drug user. But I had stopped for the past ten years before I had found out that I was HIV-positive, and I contracted it through unprotected sex from a male that knew he had it. So, it was hard for me to digest it after being an intravenous drug user for so long, being tested every year, and still coming up not positive, 'til finally after being in the drug program for two years, finding out that I was positive. It was really crazy. So, I talked to my doctor, and I was going through—I cried and cried and cried and didn't know—I wanted to die. I wanted to go and hunt him down. I wanted to beat him up and all this old kind of stuff; and I had to hold on to God and finding peace

just in the midst of, look I have it; the doctor's telling me you don't have to die with it; you can live with it, so I had to.

Hailey elaborated and described her first disclosure experiences, along with her struggle to live more openly to fulfill her desire to one day become a public speaker about HIV:

I think it took me after like ninety days of not believing that I actually had it before I sat down and really opened up and talked to a doctor concerning it. Before I even told any of my family members, I spoke to my doctor, yes. Then, afterward, I disclosed it to my mom, and my mom said—she wasn't like bent out of shape about it, but she couldn't believe it and said, 'Well, you're my daughter in spite of what you have.' My mother was very supportive, but the thing that I deal with now with having it is being open to the public because I know this is a detrimental thing that people need to be aware. People need to be tested.

After her initial disclosures, Hailey continued to disclose to more members of her family. However, Hailey described how she couldn't tell her current lover:

It's been gradual, over the years. It's been gradual, just sitting and talking with them. My sister, both of my daughters know. Basically, my whole family, yeah, they know. I was in fear of being rejected, but my family is a pretty loving family. My family was very supportive, yeah. [However], knowing that I can't afford my own place on my own, it prohibits me from just going forth and saying [to my lover], 'Look, this is it; this is how it is.' He's my sole supporter; he's the house I live in, and the car that I drive and all these things; and knowing that I can't afford my own place on my own, and fear of that I'm not gonna have a home; or I'm not gonna have a car to drive; or I'm not even gonna have a relationship, you know, so that's part of it for me.

Salena

Salena, who identifies as Puerto Rican, learned she was living with HIV in 2013 when she was pregnant with her daughter. After having her baby girl, Salena suffered postpartum depression. Now, Salena credits her daughter for saving her life and for being the reason she is not homeless. Salena recalled some of her initial disclosures and the support she received from her older sister and brother:

I told my sister first, and the way I told her was, 'Don't tell my brother!' 'cause I was embarrassed to actually tell a male, like my brother. [When I told my sister], it went okay. My sister was supportive, of course, even though she blamed it on my baby father, which is the person that gave me the virus, but I didn't want to

> blame him per se. I was explaining it to her. It is what it is. That I have this HIV virus, and this is my life. At first, I wanted to tell my family, of course. Well, [my sister] told my brother, which I didn't want that to happen. And he was like, 'No matter what, I'm still your brother, and I still love you.' After I told my sister and my brother, I told a couple of friends from the church 'cause at first when I was diagnosed, I was homeless. Right now, I still have my apartment 'cause, thank God, my daughter helped me with that. I told friends from church—the pastor—and then I slowly told my other family, like my aunts and my cousins. Then, my father, but my father wasn't really too happy—of course he wasn't happy—and I had to explain to him [that] I have to take my medication. It will still be okay as far as living with the virus, but he didn't understand; so right now, I'm not really talking to my father yet 'cause I don't want him to keep telling me, 'I told you to be careful.' over and over again. So, I don't want to hear too much negative from him.

The next chapter first summarizes prior research on models of HIV disclosure. Then, drawing from my research data on HIV disclosure, I offer a new model of HIV disclosure that incorporates the concept of private and public spheres and the idea of a disclosure continuum to depict how disclosures change over time.

Chapter 2

Disclosure Research

Deciding to disclose your HIV-positive status to other people often causes anxiety. A woman needs to decide when to disclose, how to disclose, how much to disclose, and who to disclose to. This chapter first discusses three different models of the HIV disclosure process. Then, a model of HIV disclosure that incorporates the concept of a disclosure continuum is offered.

THREE MODELS OF HIV DISCLOSURE

As part of the process of disclosing, women often engage in similar steps to prepare for and conduct the disclosure. Qiao et al. (2013) identified three models of HIV disclosure used by parents to disclose to their children. The simplest model is the Four-Phase Model (Qiao et al., 2013), which is based on the theory of disease progression that hypothesizes a person is more likely to disclose to others as their disease progresses. The Four-Phase Model consists of the following stages: (1) secrecy, where the person does not want to disclose, (2) exploratory, where the person considers the possibility of disclosing, (3) readiness, where the person begins to develop a plan to disclose, and (4) disclosure, where the person discloses (Qiao et al., 2013).

The second model, the Disclosure Decision-Making Model, consists of a flowchart of decision options and goal considerations that may or may not lead to a disclosure. This model was developed and researched by Greene et al. (2012), Omarzu (2000), and Qiao et al. (2013). The Disclosure Decision-Making Model is also based on the theory of disease progression, with social influence and consequence theories added, where a person will consider the consequences of their disclosure and how their disclosure will affect others. Using the Disclosure Decision-Making Model, a person considers the breadth, duration, and depth of each disclosure. People also consider how that disclosure will affect their social status and the possible results of the disclosure (Greene et al., 2012; Omarzu, 2000; Qiao et al., 2013).

Developed by Chaudoir and Fisher (2010), Chaudoir et al. (2011), and Qiao et al. (2013), the Disclosure Processes Model is the most extensive of the three disclosure models reviewed by Qiao et al. (2013). The Disclosure Processes Model is based on social exchange theory, especially the idea of social penetration, where every interaction in a relationship prompts the analysis of immediate, future, and cumulative rewards (Altman & Taylor, 1973). Applying social exchange theory, the Disclosure Processes Model suggests people with approach goals, such as strengthening relationships and educating others, will benefit from disclosures more than individuals with avoidance goals, such as avoiding conflict and rejection in relationships.

Furthermore, Chaudoir et al. (2011) determined people living with HIV are more prone to adopt avoidance goals if they live in social contexts where there is greater cultural stigma associated with HIV, which reduces opportunities for positive responses. Using the Disclosure Processes Model, a woman considers approach and avoidance goals, available mediating processes, and possible long-term outcomes. Each disclosure event generates a feedback loop, which affects future disclosures, resulting in either more visibility or more concealment. Using these disclosure models as a foundation, the next section builds on these models and incorporates the ideas of a disclosure continuum and the concepts of private and public sphere disclosures.

THE DISCLOSURE CONTINUUM

From my interviews and research, I developed a new model of the process of disclosing HIV to others, which involves ever-widening circles as a woman discloses to more people, as illustrated in figure 2.1.

Each woman moves through this disclosure process in her own unique way, as clarified by Tamara, who emphasized, "You're unique in your disclosure. Remember there's a continuum of disclosure and wherever you fit on that continuum is okay." However, my research did uncover some commonalities that occur during private and public disclosures, which are discussed next.

PRIVATE AND PUBLIC SPHERE DISCLOSURES

A person's private sphere usually consists of their immediate family members, close friends, and sexual partners. People must balance their privacy needs with their openness needs, which requires them to continuously negotiate between their private and public spheres (Allen et al., 2012; Charmaz, 1991; Habermas, 1996). A woman's public sphere may consist of her healthcare providers, her extended family, her employer, her social media contacts, and

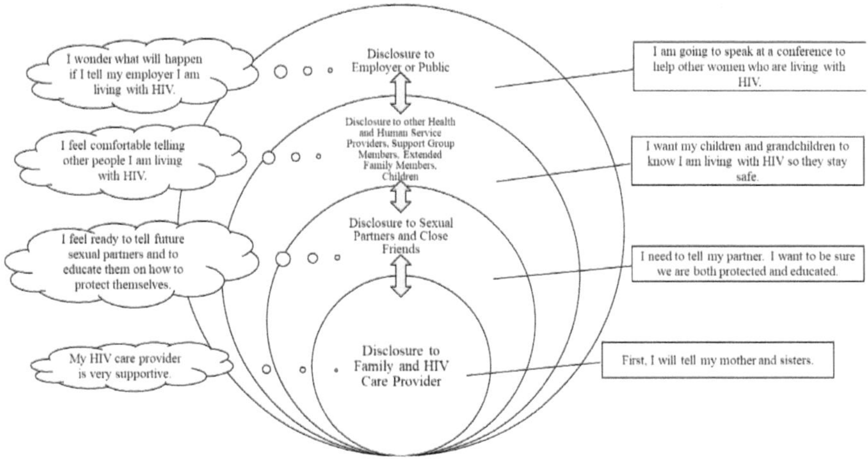

Figure 2.1. Model of HIV Disclosure (D'Amore, 2019)

possibly the public. As a woman discloses her positive status to others, her private and public spheres get blended, resulting in a disclosure continuum where private information is shared in the public sphere. A woman living with HIV must decide which people she wants to disclose her positive status to and the depth and breadth of each disclosure. For instance, in some situations, a woman needs to make a disclosure decision with little time to contemplate her choices. At other times, a situation may allow her to consider the pros and cons of disclosure and to seek the advice and support of other people.

One example of this balancing act between the private and public spheres was expressed by Destiny, who asserted, "My circle was bigger, so everybody wanted to know what was wrong with me." Ava also expressed the relief she feels after disclosing to someone, "It's like a weight is lifted off your shoulder 'cause you like, I'm sharing myself again with a person';cause sometimes HIV can take that sharing part of you away 'cause you don't wanna share yourself sometimes." This negotiation and balancing between the private and public spheres are based on each woman's analysis of the benefits and costs of disclosing in each situation.

Furthermore, after disclosing to individuals in their private spheres, women often engage in transitional disclosures that fall between the private and public spheres. These transitional disclosures could be to confidants who are in the public sphere but who are trusted by women, such as a pastor, a medical care provider, a case manager, or a church member. Transitional disclosures give women an opportunity to test disclosing their HIV-positive status in a more public way. If these transitional disclosures are met with a feeling of success, then women may disclose in a more public manner.

In the next sections, research findings and examples are given of women making private sphere disclosures, transitional disclosures, and public sphere disclosures.

Private Sphere Disclosures

Women often decide to first disclose to immediate family members, especially their mothers and sisters, since that is where loving and trusting relationships often exist (Ciambrone, 2003; D'Amore, 2019; Kidd & Clay, 2003). Even though women often find it difficult to disclose their positive status to their children and grandchildren, Ciambrone (2003) found children can also be a source of support and motivation for women. Hailey's comments illustrate this well: "Now I've went through a complacency point in my life where I said, 'I ain't taking no medication; just let me die.' I've went there. I went there, and then I said, 'I have children. I have ten grandkids. I still have a reason to live. If not for me, then for those that's coming up behind me.'"

Deciding when and how to disclose to their sexual partners is another dilemma women must contemplate in their relationships. According to Serovich et al. (2012), women often disclose to their current and past sexual partners more quickly than to other social network members. Additionally, Moskowitz and Roloff (2012) determined women employ a variety of techniques to disclose to their sexual partners with direct, verbal disclosure being the most popular method. However, sometimes women employ an indirect disclosure approach, especially if they fear rejection, stigma, or violence. An example of this cautious approach is illustrated by Ava's description of how she often disclosed her positive status to sexual partners, "I told them there may be a chance that I have HIV from a previous partner; I'm not sure. So once the relationship started, we started getting into the relationship, then I took them to the doctor with me; but I told them that there may be a chance, so that gave them a chance to say—I didn't give them a total option during that time, and I feel kind of bad about it; but I thought that was safer for me with the lifestyle and the things that I was doing and how I was living."

Another illustration of how a woman's confidence disclosing to her sexual partners changes throughout her disclosure continuum was described by Kendra, who compared her early disclosures to her later ones. Kendra related, "I didn't tell [my partner] until after we had intercourse, and that's one of the ones that I said kept having oral sex with me. I was just proud of myself for being able to open up and tell 'em." In contrast, in recent years, Kendra shared her disclosure as, "My fiancé, I told him before we even kissed because I didn't want that on my conscience." Gradually, Kendra became more comfortable disclosing to sexual partners, indicative of movement along the disclosure continuum.

As women become more comfortable disclosing their HIV-positive status to members of their private sphere, they often start to disclose more publicly, moving to a stage of transitional disclosures along the disclosure continuum.

Transitional Disclosures

A woman often continues to disclose her positive status to other people who are beyond her private sphere. These people may include her HIV specialist, her case manager, her clergyperson, her church congregation, her coworkers, her employer, and her support group. These transitional disclosures permit a woman to build her confidence in disclosing her positive status and to increase her circle of supportive others. Some women also begin to speak publicly about living with HIV, as shared by Ava: "[In the beginning], when I spoke, it was like at little rehabs or maybe I'd go show up at a march, but I wasn't the one speaking on that march; I was just there to have some information, pass out flyers. [Now] I've spoken at marches and rallies. I've spoken to classes. I've spoken at conferences."

Another example of disclosing first to a small, supportive group was reported by Nevaeh when she recalled first sharing her status with her church congregation: "Well, I actually stood up in front of the church; before I started going out to public speak, I actually stood up in front of the church and told them that I was going to be publicly speaking; so, I wanted to tell them first, and I just told them. I told them about how I got it, how long I had it; and they were very open to it."

By disclosing to small, intimate groups, women increase their confidence, practice their delivery, and receive support as they prepare to speak more publicly. They also build empathy by sharing their personal stories, as indicated by Irene's comment: "It's not out of sympathy, but empathy, but many times that is a component that people don't get a chance to hear about." Moving from private to public disclosures occurred in a variety of ways because of the diversity of possible public disclosures, such as speaking at rallies, presenting at conferences, speaking to students, posting on social media, and participating in community organizations.

Public Sphere Disclosures

To improve her ability to speak publicly, a woman often learns more about HIV to increase her knowledge and confidence to speak about HIV prevention. During interviews, participants mentioned their reason for speaking publicly about HIV prevention was their desire to educate others about the disease and ways to prevent it. For example, Nevaeh revealed her motivation to speak publicly: "I didn't want anybody else to go through that; so, this is my way of not having people go through it and trying to stop as many people as I could from getting the virus, so they wouldn't have to walk a day in my shoes. So, to me, this is my legacy that I'm leaving the world." Additionally, Josie recalled her reason for disclosing to her church congregation: "I knew there were other people there that were positive, but they didn't know how to talk about it, and so, I stood up for them."

During my interviews, the women reported the various types of public speaking and work they participate in. For example, Josie mentioned how she serves on a Patient Advisory Council and a Planning Council to help to decide how Ryan White funds will be used. Furthermore, Josie has appeared in and written several newspaper articles. Josie elaborated on her public speaking efforts: "I've gone to middle schools; I've gone to high schools; I've gone to colleges, universities; I've gone to churches; I've gone to senior centers; I've gone to senior housing. I've gone just about any place I'm asked because I think it's important to get the information out." Similarly, Nevaeh recognized the places she speaks publicly: "We've had an AIDS ministry now for about seven years. I talk to church groups; I talk to youth groups; I talk to pretty much—I've talked to groups of doctors; I've talked to medical students. I talk to the whole gamut of people. I've been in magazines. I actually was part of a documentary [about HIV]."

To prepare to speak publicly, women often gathered support and networked with other women who were living with HIV. Tamara illustrated the benefits of social networking in the following way: "Finding common ground is very important for women. It helps connect that common thread. To be in the same room with women and hear someone tell their story and like, oh, that's my story too; and you'll find out that you have a lot of common threads amongst women who live with HIV, and you need to meet those women and hear those stories." Ava also revealed the benefits she receives from her social network: "I have other women that I've never even met that I talk to, and we share; Facebook, Instagram—if it's nothing but a picture like—this is what I look like today. This is what I look like today; did you take your meds? It's that connection. We have never personally met each other, but we check on each other."

Additionally, some of the women shared how a supportive workplace increased their positive sense of self and empowered them to speak publicly. Ava's response illustrates this best: "I have great coworkers. My coworkers are my family. They are my strength. I got this [position] from coming here, volunteering, spending time, because they're open about speaking about and talking about it. It's not a shameful thing. They know the sky's not gonna fall once you say I'm HIV-positive."

The social capital built from the support given by family, friends, medical and human service providers, and supportive work environments was important for the women as they prepared for future disclosures, especially speaking publicly about living with HIV. This social network may also lead to new opportunities, as described by Nevaeh: "The pastor that I have now, she had seen a newspaper article before I even joined her church that I had did; and so, of course, she called me because then she had friends and things that had died of HIV and AIDS, and she wanted to know how to get involved. And so, she got involved, and then, I joined her church; and we started an AIDS ministry."

In the next chapter, disclosure advice is offered by the women interviewed.

Chapter 3

Disclosure Guidance from Lived Experiences

The women who I interviewed offered many different reasons for deciding to disclose in some situations and deciding not to disclose in other situations. These reasons often depended on which stage of their disclosure continuum they were at. Some of the reasons were based on approach goals, such as sharing their positive status with a possible sexual partner to negotiate safe sex. Other times, women offered their rationale for not disclosing in a situation because they didn't want to be stigmatized or lose employment. This chapter offers some of the reasons the participants gave for disclosing and not disclosing. After that, some possible benefits and costs of HIV disclosure are discussed. Finally, the participants offer advice for various types of disclosure to help guide other women who are living with HIV along their unique disclosure continuum.

DISCLOSURE RATIONALE

A woman's reasons for disclosure fluctuate along the disclosure continuum and over her life. Right after an HIV diagnosis, women usually disclose to their family and friends for support. For example, Destiny clarified her reason for telling her daughter less than a month after her HIV-positive diagnosis: "I did it for support. She was very supportive." Disclosing to family members and friends for support illustrates self-focused reasons and approach goals according to Derlega et al. (2004). These types of private sphere disclosures to intimate, trusted others also spotlight the crucial need of supportive social networks for people living with a chronic illness (Ciambrone, 2003; Foster & Gaskins, 2009).

As women begin to accept their HIV diagnosis, they usually share their positive status with their sexual partner for the reason of protection. Serovich et al. (2012) concluded women's reasons to disclose to their sexual partners included a desire to protect partners and to encourage partners to be tested for HIV. For instance, Salena reported during her interview: "I'm in a new relationship now, so I shared it with my new boyfriend. When we were getting ready to start intercourse, I had to tell him, you know." Salena's decision to disclose to her partner indicates her desire to protect him and herself as they consider having sexual intercourse. After a woman has disclosed to her family, friends, and sexual partners, she often considers sharing her positive status with others in the public, especially to educate them about HIV.

The decision to move into the public sphere to educate others about HIV often stems from a woman's faith and desire to impact the world. Nevaeh revealed her motivation as a desire to leave a legacy:

> For me, what it was, is—I sat around for about five, six years pretty much waiting to die 'cause, of course, when you have HIV, you think you're gonna die; and one day, I just said, 'You know what? I wanna leave a legacy!' And so, I wanted to know how to get involved; and I didn't want people to go through what I went through because when I found out that I had it, it was just, 'You got it! You're gonna die! That's it!' There was no education around it. In '89, they didn't educate you; and as an African American female living with it, you didn't get educated.

Similarly, Josie expounded on her rationale for deciding to publicly disclose her positive status to educate others:

> Some of it's personality; some of it's upbringing. Because I come from a very strong faith-based family, so I was always taught you never say why me, you say why not me; and I was taught that if you have faith in God, He has ordained everything that's gonna happen to you anyway. There's a reason. Now, you can sit around and mope and be negative, or you can look for the positive side and step up and do what you have to do. And so, having been brought up with that embedded in my head, I never felt down or negative about it.

On the other side of the disclosure continuum, there are varying degrees of nondisclosure. In the next section, the women I interviewed share their reasons for deciding not to disclose their HIV-positive status to others.

NONDISCLOSURE RATIONALE

From my research, the reasons for nondisclosure often appeared to be based on misperceptions, fear, and a lack of support. For example, Kendra revealed why she was reluctant to disclose to her family: "I don't wanna be a burden 'cause I'm a very independent person. I don't wanna be a burden on them. I don't want them to pity me, things like that." Kendra went on to express why she especially didn't want to disclose to her mother: "One of the reasons why I won't tell my mother—because she's in her eighties. Number one, I don't wanna worry her. That's the biggest thing. But originally, I didn't tell her because I didn't want to—she was not informed. She didn't have any education about HIV and AIDS; so, her first reaction was gonna be like what society would do back in that day. Paper plates, paper cups, watching everything you're doing; and that's an uncomfortable feeling, so I didn't wanna go through that."

Kendra's reasons for nondisclosure are based on her feeling she would be a burden to her family and that her family may see her as a burden because she is living with HIV. Additionally, Kendra fears her mother's reaction to her HIV-positive status. Some women also fear the loss of support, or even violence, from sexual partners. Therefore, they choose not to disclose their positive status to their significant others.

Another type of nondisclosure occurs in places of employment. Although the Americans with Disabilities Act of 1990 (ADA) identified HIV as a protected disability (Americans with Disabilities Act, 1990; U.S. Department of Justice, 2008), many people living with HIV are reluctant to inform their employers because they fear discrimination and may not be aware of their legal rights as protected by the ADA (Timmons & Fesko, 2004). Deciding to disclose HIV to an employer involves considering the nature of the work environment, the risk of disclosure, the desire for privacy, the consequences of disclosing, and the consequences of not disclosing (Fesko, 2001). For instance, Josie recommended: "No, I wouldn't tell [an employer], you know, unless you sick or something; otherwise, they can't look at you and tell you sick. Ain't nobody's business." Nevaeh concurred with Josie's advice when she cautioned, "So, if it's a situation that you don't have to disclose, I don't feel you should. If you wanted maybe to disclose to your supervisor or something, just because if you get sick or something—I think you have to be very careful with that."

In the next section, the women I interviewed share some of the positive and negative results from their disclosures.

POSITIVE RESULTS OF DISCLOSURES

The women who I interviewed reported some of the positive results that came from disclosing their HIV-positive status to others. First, each of the participants expressed how they received support from others after disclosing their status. This support was especially important after their initial diagnosis. The women also spoke about how they gained acceptance from others after disclosing. For example, Michelle recalled the positive reactions of her friends after they learned of her positive status: "I told several of my male friends, and they are all positive. They were all like, 'And? So what?' They stayed my friends, and I still talk to them; and those were people that I met in the recovery process of the drug addiction and the ladies in my building; we all came through the same drug treatment, and now, we all have apartments in the same building; and they're just fine with it. And I've had two relationships, sexual relationships; they didn't care either. They were like, 'And what? We all got something.'"

Some of the women spoke about how their disclosures brought them comfort beyond the support and acceptance they received. For instance, Ava reported the benefits she gets from disclosing her HIV-positive status to others: "It's a freeing experience to share that part of you again with people, and after you said it, can't nobody hold it against you anymore. Sometimes, disclosing can become an outer body experience. You look down, and be like, 'Why did I do that? I can't take it back now.' Or 'Oh my God! I'm so glad it went good! Oh, thank you!' You're just overjoyed that it went even better than you expected and that gives you a boost. That gives everybody's confidence level a boost—even without having the virus."

Tamara described the benefits she gains from speaking publicly about HIV, "For me, [sharing my story] helps my process and the process of helping other women living with HIV because I am an educator. It gave me a positive impact to share with other people. And I think it helps other people who are newly diagnosed to hear from women who've been living with it for a long time and see their journey; that their journey's a positive one, and their journey as they move forward will be a positive one as well."

NEGATIVE RESULTS OF DISCLOSURES

Alternatively, some disclosures result in more negative outcomes in which women do not find support, comfort, or acceptance. Some disclosures result in hurt feelings, rejection, discrimination, and stigma. One example of disclosures of this type are unsanctioned disclosures, where someone takes confidential information that was shared with them and informs other people without permission. For instance, Tamara recalled an unsanctioned disclosure experience: "[My baby sister] felt like she should go tell my son about my status without my permission. I was angry. I was disappointed because I felt like I'm the one that should do that, and then, when I got the chance to tell my sixteen-year-old son about my status, he was hurt, not so much of the fact that I was living with HIV, he was hurt because he should've heard it first from me and not from someone else."

Social media has expanded the opportunity for unsanctioned disclosures, as illustrated by Salena's experience soon after her diagnosis:

> So right after I told [my baby's father] his female cousin, she blast it on Facebook. Yeah, even though I wanted to tell everybody on Facebook about my diagnosis and my disclosure, but my therapist decided not to do it yet. So, I agreed with my therapist, but right after she said it; the way she said it was, 'Make sure you take your HIV medication.' On a comment, and I'm like, 'Oh my goodness! What happened if somebody read that comment?' So finally, when I disclosed it on Facebook or social media, I was like, oh my God, it's not a big thing. As of right after I disclosed it, it was really supportive.

Some women also experience rejection after disclosing their positive status to others. Rejection was especially detrimental in the workplace, as illustrated by Nevaeh as she recalled, "I actually lost a job because I disclosed. I was working in a nursing home, and I was working as an activities assistant; and I was really just doing activities with the clients; and then, at lunchtime, I would cut up their food, but when I told them that I had it, they stopped me from cutting up the peoples' food; and then they told me they'd fire me, and they really made—they never gave me a reason, because they didn't have a reason, so I knew it was because of my HIV status."

Based on their lived experiences disclosing their positive status to their families, friends, healthcare providers, employers, and the public, interview participants next offer some guidance to other women as they contemplate disclosing their status to others.

DISCLOSURE GUIDANCE

One of the key recommendations given by interview participants was to be selective when deciding to disclose positive status to others. Tamara recommends, "Examine why you're disclosing, who you're disclosing to, and where you're disclosing at." Laila concurred with this advice, stating, "Before you disclose, make sure that that is what you wanna do. Be sure that you're ready for that. Be sure that you're ready to take on the stigmatism that comes with it because we still have people out here that's so ignorant to the fact, that are not educated on it. So, prepare yourself."

Another disclosure recommendation was to be careful and safe when disclosing HIV-positive status to others. Ava suggested, "Ask for help. Write down what you're gonna say to somebody." Additionally, Destiny advised:

"Discretion. It's not everybody's business. The best way to do it is to feel a person out. Have a conversation about HIV. See if they're phobic. Then, you decide whether you wanna tell them that or not."

Tamara offered her recommendation when disclosing to sexual partners: "It was the first thing after we dated and talked about is to disclose my status to him and give him the opportunity know about this—this about your health, too. You wanna be in this relationship, this is what it is, right, and how I can keep you safe, and you can even keep each other safe when we talk about transmission of any kind of viruses." Furthermore, Kendra revealed her experience disclosing to sexual partners: "The more you do it, it gets easier. You begin to not care about the reaction, and you can sleep at night knowing you disclosed it versus being intimate with someone and not disclosing it."

Some general guidance from the women I interviewed came from Tamara, who gave her advice to other women as they prepare to disclose their positive status: "Everyone has their own process of disclosure." Irene said that disclosure is "an individual choice because once you say something it's out there, and you can't retract that." Destiny cautioned that disclosure "is a very personal issue, and be careful who you disclose to, simply because some people will use it against you. Some people will use it to hurt you." Finally, Nevaeh shared her thoughts: "I think before you disclose your status, you have got to be okay with your status first because, like I said earlier, when you disclose, you cannot take it back."

Combining the insights I gained from my interviews with prior research on HIV disclosure, I compiled some of the characteristics of the phenomenon of HIV disclosure. Chapter 4 details the phenomenon of HIV disclosure and describes the components of the lived experience of HIV disclosure.

Chapter 4

The Phenomenology of HIV Disclosure

To develop the phenomenology of HIV disclosure, I combined my qualitative data results and applied Seidman's (2013) concept of forming lived experiences with the components of lived time, lived space, lived human relationships, and lived body. Figure 4.1 depicts a possible model of the phenomenon of HIV disclosure.

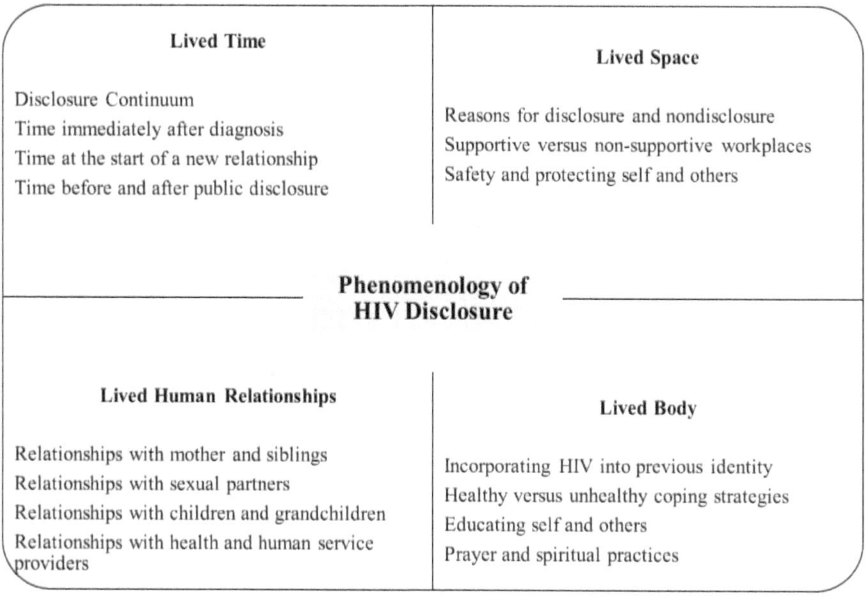

Figure 4.1. Phenomenology of HIV Disclosure (D'Amore, 2019)

LIVED TIME

The lived time component of the phenomenon of HIV disclosure consists of the disclosure continuum, which evolves from the time of diagnosis to public speaking. Lived time also focuses on the timing of private sphere disclosures and the occurrences of public sphere disclosures. Additionally, a person's lived time relates to their age at diagnosis and their time living with HIV. Furthermore, lived time consists of the time in society a person lives in. For instance, the experience of living with HIV was vastly different during the 1980s as compared to now.

LIVED SPACE

As a woman decides whether to disclose to others, she must consider the lived space she is in. Lived space refers to where a woman lives, where she works, the community and society she lives in, and her interaction with this space. If the lived space is a supportive setting where trust exists, a woman is more prone to share her positive status. On the other hand, if a woman is in a space where she fears the reaction of others to her disclosure, she will be unlikely to disclose.

This lived space may be represented in several ways. For example, some interview participants shared how supportive their workplaces were because they worked for organizations focused on HIV care services. However, other women reported their workplace disclosures resulted in a loss of employment. Lived space is also illustrated by women who choose to speak publicly about their experiences of living with HIV to educate others about HIV prevention. By speaking about their experiences, these public speakers help to change the lived space of their communities. The disclosure of positive status also affects a woman's lived human relationships as discussed next.

LIVED HUMAN RELATIONSHIPS

Each disclosure affects a woman's human relationships with her family, friends, and sexual partners. Sometimes, she will experience rejection. More often, a woman receives support from her family, friends, and sexual partners. The social support women receive from their family, friends, and sexual partners help them to live a meaningful life with HIV. A strong support system is especially important as a woman discloses positive status in public. Furthermore, disclosures affect human relationships by either strengthening them and increasing trust or weakening them because of fear and stigma. Lived human relationships built on love, compassion, understanding, and empathy are vital to sustaining HIV endurance.

LIVED BODY

When a woman is living with HIV, she often educates herself and others about HIV's effects on the body. For example, as a woman becomes more educated about HIV, she is then able to educate her sexual partners and family members. Additionally, as a woman speaks publicly, she often continues to educate herself about HIV prevention, so she is prepared to share her lived experience with others.

The lived body also refers to how living with HIV affects a woman's sexual life, her decisions regarding pregnancy, her identity, and society's view of her. As a woman ages with HIV, her lived body experiences change over time because she often encounters additional health concerns that compound the effects of HIV.

Applying the concept of the phenomenology of HIV disclosure with the concept of a disclosure continuum, figure 4.2 depicts a possible timeline of HIV disclosure for women who are living with HIV.

Because each woman's lived time, lived space, lived human relationships, and lived body are unique to her life and circumstances, the components of this model will vary. Furthermore, because of the uniqueness of each woman's disclosure continuum, women do not move along the continuum in the same way, and often, they do not disclose beyond the people in their

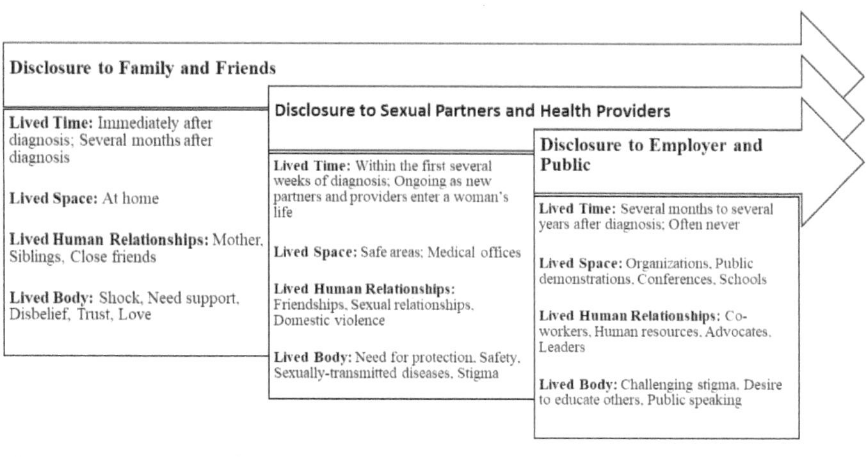

Figure 4.2. Timeline of HIV Disclosure (D'Amore, 2019)

private sphere. I now offer my personal connection to the lived experience of HIV disclosure and four key takeaways to remember about HIV disclosure to conclude section one.

Personal Connection

My Lived Experience with HIV Disclosure

In this section, I will apply the components of a lived experience of HIV disclosure as I have experienced them. I hope this section helps to further illustrate the components of lived time, lived space, lived human relationships, and lived body as they apply to HIV disclosure.

MY LIVED TIME

Having lived with HIV since 1998, I have observed how my disclosure decisions have evolved over time. When I was first diagnosed with HIV, I did not want to tell anyone because I was ashamed and embarrassed that I had not used safer sex practices with my partner. I blamed myself for contracting HIV and for not protecting myself. I especially did not want to tell my immediate family because I thought they would judge me and criticize my actions. The only people I felt comfortable disclosing to initially were a male friend, my HIV specialist, my sexual partner, and anonymous others who I spoke to over the telephone and who staffed helplines for people living with HIV.

When Susan, my HIV specialist, asked me to speak publicly with her to educate others about women's experiences with HIV, I adamantly refused her offer initially. I declared there was no way I wanted to speak to anyone about living with HIV. However, when she delineated the benefits other women and healthcare providers would gain from hearing about my lived experiences, I reconsidered and added I would try it. After I spoke a couple of times in public, I decided I had to tell my immediate family members because I did not want them to hear about it from others. Slowly, over time, I disclosed to my immediate family and to my close friends.

Then, I started dating, and with each date, I had to decide when to disclose my positive status. From my first conversations with a prospective partner, I was thinking about when and how to tell him I was HIV-positive. I usually waited until the relationship started to get more serious before disclosing, but I would tell my partner before we engaged in sex. Each time I disclosed my positive status, I braced myself for my partner's reaction. Some partners left the relationship after finding out, while other partners wanted to continue our relationship. With each disclosure, I realized you cannot control how other people react when they hear you are HIV-positive. I learned to accept the other person's reaction and not take it personally. Over time, I became more comfortable disclosing my positive status to others both in the private and public spheres.

MY LIVED SPACE

Over the years, I have been fortunate to be able to disclose my HIV-positive status in safe, supportive spaces. I was often able to plan where and when I was going to disclose. I also mentally practiced what I was going to say and how I was going to say it. Additionally, I thought about how the other person might react to my disclosure and possible ways to mitigate a negative reaction. I always tried to have some educational materials to offer to people, and I prepared myself to answer their questions.

I usually have disclosed to others in a face-to-face conversation. These conversations have often occurred in my home or in the home of the other person. I have sometimes disclosed over the telephone, which allowed me to put some physical space between the other person and myself. This disclosure option was especially useful if I thought strong emotions would result from my disclosure. Sometimes, I have disclosed through writing. My written disclosures have most often occurred on medical intake forms and to employers. While people are often surprised when they learn that I am living with HIV, I have been fortunate to not experience significant discrimination because of my positive status.

MY LIVED HUMAN RELATIONSHIPS

Listening to the disclosure experiences of others, I again realize how fortunate I am. When I disclosed my HIV-positive status to my immediate family and friends, they all responded with love and support. I feared they would blame and judge me, but they did not. Their compassionate responses helped me to resolve the shame and blame I placed on myself. Also, when I have disclosed to sexual partners, I have been fortunate they have mostly reacted with composure. I know other women who have experienced anger, blame, and rejection after disclosing to their partners. Additionally, when I disclosed to others, my relationships often became more intimate and strengthened by my willingness to be vulnerable and share a private part of myself. Because my disclosures have generated mostly positive responses, I am more prone to disclose to others in the future.

MY LIVED BODY

When I first discovered I was living with HIV, I was physically weak from the virus' impact on my body. My physical weakness and the possibility of being admitted to a hospital motivated me to disclose to my parents and siblings. I didn't want them to learn of my positive status from a medical provider at a hospital. Luckily, after I started taking the antiretroviral medications, my physical strength came back, and I could take my time before telling my family.

Disclosing my positive status to my family was very difficult because I felt ashamed and blamed myself for becoming HIV-positive. Through heavy sobs, I shared my devastating news with them and was astonished by their love, compassion, and forgiveness. Their generous responses helped me to move along my journey toward forgiving myself and lifting the burdens of blame and shame I was carrying.

When I spoke publicly with Susan and Christine, I was always very nervous before I spoke. However, while speaking, I reminded myself about the importance of my message and the need to educate others about HIV. By speaking publicly about HIV, I hoped I was helping to reduce HIV stigma in society. The best part about these presentations was getting to see and speak to Christine. I drew inspiration from her as I learned more about her HIV journey. Becoming friends with Christine showed me the importance of a social support network of women living with HIV who can openly share their experiences with each other and who can foster HIV endurance through their shared experiences of disclosure.

Four Key Takeaways

HIV Disclosure

- There's a disclosure continuum, and wherever you are on the continuum is okay because everyone has their own disclosure process.
- Disclosure is an individual choice, so carefully consider the consequences of a disclosure and be in a safe and supportive space when you disclose.
- Private sphere disclosures include intimate others such as family, friends, and sexual partners, while transitional disclosures help prepare people to disclose in the public sphere, which includes disclosure to employers, healthcare providers, and the public.
- Support groups, case managers, and HIV specialists can help women prepare for and reflect on their disclosure experiences through education and discussion of disclosure results.

SECTION II

HIV Stigma

Chapter 5

Experiences of Stigma

The women I interviewed revealed the stigmatizing attitudes and behaviors they sometimes received from their family members, lovers, healthcare providers, and employers. This chapter summarizes my findings based on the interviews I conducted. Chapter 6 bolsters my findings by offering research on the effects of marginalization and intersectionality on women's experiences of HIV stigma and the effects of HIV stigma, especially on older women living with HIV. To conclude this section, chapter 7 offers suggestions on ways to challenge HIV stigma at the micro, meso, and macro levels of society.

HIV STIGMA FROM LOVED ONES

Stigma often appears after a person living with HIV discloses their status to a loved one. For example, Nichole, who is a white woman in her fifties, shared the stigma she experienced from family members. After Nichole and her husband tested positive for HIV in 1992, they informed their parents and siblings. While their parents accepted the news, Nichole's husband's siblings became "just kind of standoffish" and "He had a brother and sister that wouldn't even come around us." Nichole also recalled, "My grandmother started putting names on glasses and stuff."

Some interview participants feared their loved ones' reactions and chose not to disclose. For instance, Hailey revealed the stigma her lover expressed as the reason for her nondisclosure: "Living in a household with my significant other saying that he wish he could line all the HIV infected and all the gay people up and just shoot 'em down; so it kind a like prohibits me from being open and honest with him with what's going on."

Other women expressed the stigma they experienced at the community and societal levels, especially early in the AIDS pandemic. Ava gave her opinion about the persistence of HIV stigma in communities of color:

"Stigma continues because Black people have a culture that promotes keeping information private and religious taboos on speaking about sex and HIV." Additionally, Tamara recalled her experience living with HIV in the 1990s: "I come from an area where AIDS was talked about in a whisper. Even doctors and providers were saying AIDS in a very low voice because they didn't say it out loud because they wasn't sure what it was." While the treatment of HIV has progressed tremendously since the start of antiretroviral treatments, interview participants still encountered stigma when interacting with healthcare providers beyond their HIV specialist, as discussed next.

HIV STIGMA IN HEALTHCARE

As I mentioned in my preface, I experienced some HIV stigma at the beginning of my HIV journey when I went for my chest X-ray. Often, I was most vulnerable to experiencing stigma when I went to a new healthcare provider. For example, in February 2000, I went to a new gynecologist. After I revealed to him that I was living with HIV, he completed my pap test. Then, he handed me seven sample packs of birth control pills and advised, "Whatever you do, don't get pregnant." Without another word, he walked out the door. Another example of stigma was when I went to a new primary care provider in October 2001. She questioned me several different ways trying to determine if I had a history of drug use. I kept answering that I never used intravenous drugs. Exasperated by my answers, she exclaimed, "Well, how did you get HIV?" I explained I was infected through unprotected sexual intercourse. The doctor shook her head and blurted, "What a pity!"

In 2002, I was able to reconnect with my original HIV specialist, Susan, who was able to care for my primary care needs as well as my HIV needs because she was a certified nurse practitioner. Susan recommended a gynecologist who worked with other women living with HIV, and I was able to receive excellent and nonjudgmental care from him. Since 2002, I have been fortunate to receive my healthcare needs in settings that are more accepting of people living with HIV.

Similarly, interview participants talked about the wonderful healthcare they received, especially from their HIV specialist. However, they also shared some of the stigmatizing behaviors and attitudes they encountered while trying to obtain healthcare. For instance, Nichole reported some painful experiences she and her husband had with medical providers in the 1990s: "One time, my husband and I went to a dental appointment, and they kept us waiting for two hours. They never did see us. Another time, my husband was in the hospital, and the nurses would leave my husband's food out in the hallway and not tell him his food was out there. They would just—you could hear 'em fighting over who was gonna go in the room."

Another example was given by Irene when she was seeking medical care and instead received HIV stigma:

> I went to have carpal tunnel surgery on one of my hands one time, and again, I was very honest. I told the doctor I have HIV; and so, the anesthesiologist had come in, and he goes, 'Oh, I see you have HIV. How'd you get it?' And I said, 'Well sir,' I said, 'that's up to me to discuss with you if I choose to,' I said, 'but I'm not here for that. I'm not here to discuss that.' And finally, I just got up off of the table. It was just his whole demeanor, and I said, 'You know what, I don't want you touching me.' And I got up off the table and left.

A final example was communicated by Ava, who recalled her experience of HIV stigma while visiting her podiatrist and how she used it as a teachable moment:

> I've had people that didn't even want to shut the door when I was in the room; or they'd go and everybody, instead of just putting on a pair of gloves, they got on a surgical mask. I'm like, 'Well, who is that for? What is wrong?' Listen, I thought they found out something else was wrong with me. That scared me to death. Like I'm not gonna kiss you. We're not having sex. Oh, and by the way, you can't get it from kissing. So, those are teachable moments; sometimes, you had to teach providers what not to do. I know I've been around people that have been boo-hoo and crying about their experiences with the doctor, like I don't ever wanna go back to the doctor and that's not healthy or good. Doctors are people too.

I also asked interview participants about their experiences of discrimination in employment situations. They advised caution when disclosing HIV in the workplace unless it is a supportive environment. Several of the women shared the painful stigma they experienced from their employers.

HIV STIGMA AT WORK

When considering disclosing at a workplace where stigma could exist, Tamara suggests asking yourself the following: "Are you running the risk of disclosing your status, and they covering up and saying that you wasn't doing your job duties, when the real reason is that they are discriminating against you because you're HIV-positive?"

Additionally, Michelle recommends caution when considering disclosing in the workplace or in a church congregation:

> Not your job, no, because like I said, you go there, and you meet strangers. You're going there to earn money. You're not going there to pal around, so I would suggest that you not disclose it on your job or at your church, unless you know that they have an AIDS or HIV awareness group within their church. Keep that thing to yourself because you'll be ostracized. People will—in your church, people are supposed to love you—but people are people; and people have their own personal ideas about what AIDS is, 'How did you get it?' Everything is 'eww.' So, you have to be careful. You have to be careful that you don't put yourself in a place where once you tell these people, you are no longer accepted like you were yesterday. So yeah, you gotta really think it through.

Ava concurred with this advice and recounted her experiences:

> A lot of places that I had previously worked at, and they had even been with ministers, I've never disclosed and that's because I didn't wanna be prejudged. Take me on who I am, not what illness I carry. So sometimes, you see, in certain workplaces, the conversations that go on—how people say, 'I seen this, and I seen that.' They can even be talking to you not knowing that you even HIV-positive. So, you don't wanna—well, I'm not gonna say nothin' up in here; I'm just gonna get this paycheck; do what I got to do to live.

Ava elaborated, sharing, "Then, your bosses wanna talk about, 'Oh, what if she gets sick? What about medical coverage? Oh, we can't afford to take care of her for the rest of her life. We gotta figure out a way how to fire her, chase her out.' And that has been done in a lot of places, not specifically to me, but some people that I'm real close with. So, I can say it wasn't done to my person, but it was done to me 'cause being done to them is also being done to me."

This advice of not disclosing in places where stigma is anticipated to occur is a form of strategic concealment and selective disclosure that people use around loved ones, healthcare providers, and employers who they believe are not open to the idea of a person with HIV in their midst. People employ strategic concealment and selective disclosure to try to avoid HIV stigma and to try to protect themselves from experiencing HIV stigma, as described in the next section.

STRATEGIC CONCEALMENT AND SELECTIVE DISCLOSURE

One example of practicing selective disclosure was given by Frederica, an African American woman who discovered she was living with HIV in 2005. Frederica shared, "Since I found out that I had HIV, I've only told three people that I have HIV. I will never tell nobody else because people are—I don't know, it's like, I don't know. It's they're critical of, you know, the people, you know; and I hear people talk about people that they know have it, and it's negative; and I find myself being real—what's the word I'm looking for—standing up for them people, knowing that I myself have it, you know."

Furthermore, Ava revealed her way of dealing with HIV stigma during her early years before becoming a public advocate for HIV prevention: "I still wasn't going out telling people about it. I was still shaming people that had HIV, so that it would draw the attention away from me during those early years, and that's honest. I didn't wanna tell anybody."

Nevaeh reported how she handles stigma if she encounters it when obtaining medical care: "My experience has been pretty good; I guess because I'm an outgoing person. I just don't tolerate stigma in any kinda way, so thank God, I've never had experience that kinda stigma. And with doctors and things, I tell them right away. I tell them when I go to the emergency room, and I know I don't have to, but I do. And if they act like they're gonna get a little funny, I just tell them I don't want them in my room, and they need to send someone else in."

Hailey talked about how she is trying to move beyond stigma's confinement to live a more open life of acceptance:

> I feel like a heavy weight is on me because I haven't been totally honest with everybody that's around me, you understand, in fear of the stigma, in fear of what they may think. I can't be in bondage anymore concerning the minds of what people may think. Before I was alright with it, I was in fear of not having friends anymore, being isolated. I lived with being isolated a lot, still today. I isolate myself, except when I come out and go out in the street, but in my home surroundings, I'm truly isolated inside. We all face things that we don't even wanna tell nobody about.

In the next chapter, my research findings are supported by prior research on stigma, marginalization, intersectionality, and the effects of HIV stigma.

Chapter 6

HIV Stigma Research

Stigma associated with HIV is linked to three different stigmas identified by Goffman (1963). HIV stigma has components of stigma related to physical deformities, stigma related to weakness of character, and stigma related to membership in a despised social group (Goffman, 1963; Ogden & Nyblade, 2005). According to Herek (1999), people perceive a person who is living with HIV as being responsible for contracting the virus, and they also believe the person living with HIV is disrupting social interaction by putting other people at risk of contracting HIV. This belief is especially true for HIV because people perceive it as incurable and fatal (Ogden & Nyblade, 2005). Furthermore, society views people's culpability differently based on how they acquired HIV. For example, children living with HIV are seen as the least culpable. Similarly, women who were infected with HIV by their sexual partners or husbands are viewed as less guilty when compared to women infected with HIV through sex work or injection drug use (Ogden & Nyblade, 2005).

African American women are especially prone to experiencing societal separation because of marginalization and intersectionality (Collins, 1990; Crenshaw, 1994; Gilbert & Wright, 2003; Pellowski et al., 2013). Factors impacting African American women's lived experiences include socioeconomic factors, such as the lack of equal opportunities in the areas of education, employment, and housing, and personal factors, such as race, ethnicity, gender, and sexual orientation (Pellowski et al., 2013). Additional factors impacting the lives of some women include poverty, institutional racism, domestic violence, past sexual abuse, incarceration, and sexually transmitted infections (Gilbert & Wright, 2003). These factors increase the likelihood a woman living with HIV will suffer marginalization as she encounters intersectional stigma from a combination of these factors.

Women are especially vulnerable to economic factors which increase the opportunities for discrimination and marginalization. This is because women often act as primary caregivers to others. In taking on this societal role, women often struggle to meet the basic needs of food, shelter, and safety for themselves and their loved ones due to underemployment or unemployment (Farmer et al., 2011). Compounding these economic factors, women often have less access to affordable healthcare, legal protection, and inheritance according to Farmer et al. (2011), which increases their economic dependency and vulnerability to discrimination.

Additionally, as women age and go through menopause, they may encounter the intersectional stigma of ageism and HIV. According to Herron et al. (2022), many older women living with HIV face financial barriers due to changes in their family structure or employment. Older positive women may also confront limited mental and physical healthcare because of geographic locations and a lack of accessibility (Herron et al., 2022). Also, women living with HIV may suffer stigma when they seek healthcare to treat comorbidities, such as cancer, heart disease, osteoporosis, diabetes, and cognitive impairment (Herron et al., 2022). Women aging with HIV need support to manage the emotional effects resulting from the impacts of social isolation, economic disruptions, changing HIV treatment, and multiple pharmaceuticals to treat HIV and other comorbidities (Herron et al., 2022).

Unfortunately, when women seek help to manage their healthcare, financial, and emotional needs, they often encounter stigma and discrimination instead. According to Spence et al. (2022), women continue to bear HIV stigma when seeking medical care, which fosters a lack of trust of healthcare providers. From their research, Spence et al. (2022) determined some healthcare providers in Washington, D.C. still show evidence of sentiments of HIV stigma and feel uncomfortable discussing topics of safe sex, sexual history, drug use, and HIV prevention services with patients.

According to Nyblade and MacQuarrie (2006), there are four key indicators of HIV stigma. The first indicator is fear of casual transmission, such as refusing to have contact with a person who is living with HIV or requiring them to use disposable plates. The second indicator is focused on values and involves shaming, blaming, and judging a person for having contracted HIV. The third indicator is enacted stigma or discrimination, such as terminating a person's employment after finding out they are HIV-positive. The final indicator focuses on disclosure, namely how a person discloses their positive status and the effects of each disclosure (Nyblade & MacQuarrie, 2006). D'Amore (2019) found the experience of HIV stigma causes people to isolate themselves, to choose nondisclosure, and to not seek necessary medical care to mitigate the effects of HIV stigma, as discussed in the next section.

EFFECTS OF HIV STIGMA

Because a person's HIV-positive status overshadows other parts of a person's identity, the inequality resulting from race, class, and gender is compounded, according to Berger (2004). This dynamic causes poor women of color to absorb the greatest impact of HIV stigma because of their low social status (Berger, 2004). Additionally, Sandelowski et al. (2004) identified how women encounter more intense HIV stigma because of their gender. Sandelowski et al. (2004) also determined the pervasiveness of felt and enacted stigma and the continued need for stigma management to mitigate the effects of HIV stigma.

Furthermore, the effects of HIV stigma occur at the macro and micro levels of society (Rintamaki & Weaver, 2008). For example, at the macro level, HIV stigma is expressed by the laws and policies that affect the rights of people living with HIV, such as the 1987 travel ban that prevented people living with HIV from traveling to the United States until it was lifted in 2009 (amfAR, 2022). HIV stigma is also evident at the macro level in laws that criminalize the transmission or potential transmission of HIV (Lazzarini et al., 2013; Lehman et al., 2014)

At the micro level, HIV stigma occurs in relationships through the acts of rejection, isolation, and harassment. For instance, some people living with HIV have come across stigmatizing attitudes from healthcare personnel who have refused to provide care or who have employed excessive safety precautions (Rintamaki & Weaver, 2008). These forms of HIV stigma often cause a positive person to have increased stress and depression, increased guilt and shame, increased social isolation and self-rejection, and often increased risk-taking activities, such as substance abuse (Rendina et al., 2019; Rintamaki & Weaver, 2008). Due to a reduced social network, reduced mobility, reduced energy, and reduced cognitive functioning, older people living with HIV are especially susceptible to loneliness and isolation, which is exacerbated by HIV stigma (Rendina et al., 2019).

Additionally, Herron et al. (2022) described how women's healthcare and life choices are constrained by intersectional stigma connected to gender, ethnicity, and HIV. Because of their fear of encountering discrimination and HIV stigma, some women travel long distances to obtain medical care from providers with more experience caring for women who are living with HIV (Herron et al., 2022). Furthermore, as women age, their financial situation sometimes worsens as they experience higher medical costs and possible unemployment or underemployment according to Herron et al. (2022).

The next chapter focuses on ways to mitigate the effects of HIV stigma.

Chapter 7

Challenging HIV Stigma

To challenge HIV stigma at the micro, meso, and macro levels of society, positive people and their advocates can employ several strategies that have been proven effective. The micro level of society consists of an individual's relationships with family and friends. Organizations and community groups compose the meso-level of society. The macro level of society consists of the legal system, economy, and government of various nations.

MICRO LEVEL

Because stigma is a socially constructed phenomenon, a boundary is created between the stigmatized and nonstigmatized. An individual often self-categorizes and shifts from the healthy, normal group to the stigmatized group after learning they are living with HIV (Rintamaki, 2009). To manage the negative emotions that are associated with HIV stigma, such as anxiety and depression, people often practice concealing their HIV-positive status to pass as normal. Examples of selective disclosures and strategic concealments were given at the end of chapter 5. These are common methods to reduce the exposure to and the experience of HIV stigma at the micro level of society (D'Amore, 2019; Goffman, 1963; Smith et al., 2012). Deciding whether to disclose positive status often causes a person living with HIV psychological stress and anxiety because a positive person may be attempting to pass and may not have disclosed their status to others. The person may be torn between two groups: a group that is aware of their positive status and a group that is unaware (D'Amore, 2019; Goffman, 1963).

Another common strategy is to use preventative disclosure and to educate others to reduce social rejection and generate acceptance (HIV.gov., 2020). People who construct a positive meaning from their HIV diagnosis and view HIV as a catalyst for positive behavioral change often engage in more educational outreach and activism, which helps to reduce HIV stigma (HIV.gov.,

2020; Rintamaki, 2009). Additionally, by participating in support groups, engaging in collective activism, and speaking publicly about HIV prevention, individuals enhance their self-identity and develop coping strategies to mitigate the negative emotions associated with stigmatizing experiences. Through educational outreach and collective activism, people living with HIV educate the public and challenge HIV stigma in society (D'Amore, 2019; HIV.gov., 2020; Rintamaki & Weaver, 2008).

MESO-LEVEL

As people incorporate their HIV-positive status into their social identity, they help to minimize HIV stigma in various organizations at the meso-level of society. Women can do this by disclosing their positive status to others in the community organizations they participate in, or if they do not want to disclose their positive status, women can speak about HIV prevention. For example, the women I interviewed reported how they spoke to their church congregations about HIV. By speaking publicly, women help to address stigma about HIV and educate others about HIV prevention. Additionally, some interview participants disclosed their positive status to their employers. However, some employers were not receptive to this information. The women also shared their attempts to educate healthcare providers. This is especially critical because, according to Spence et al. (2022), there is still a great need for ongoing education to reduce HIV stigma in the healthcare fields.

Another way to reduce HIV stigma at the meso-level of society is by constructing social networks with other women, either in person or through social media. Through social networks, women living with HIV strengthen their social capital, educate each other, and see commonalities through their shared experiences (D'Amore, 2019). By increasing the number of support groups by and for women living with HIV, women can form networks and participate in decision-making exercises to test out various disclosure scenarios in a safe, supportive environment (D'Amore, 2019). Additionally, these support groups would provide a safe, nonjudgmental space to discuss encounters with HIV stigma and provide an opportunity to role play ways to challenge HIV stigma in various settings (D'Amore, 2019).

MACRO LEVEL

To reduce HIV stigma at the macro level, the media could be employed to produce and distribute public service announcements to educate the public about HIV and how it is transmitted. Additionally, media can be created to positively portray people who are living with HIV. Using social media and traditional forms of media, a vast number of people can be communicated with to reduce the amount of HIV stigma in society by building an understanding of and connection with people living with HIV.

To prepare for the increasing number of older adults living with HIV, Rendina et al. (2019) recommend developing a comprehensive model for long-term care that integrates the medical, dental, mental health, and substance use treatment care that older positive people need. This care could be provided in a one-stop primary care setting with trained healthcare professionals who are educated about the unique needs of older adults who are aging with HIV. Additionally, Lau-Ng et al. (2020) recommend geriatric training for staff who work at long-term care facilities to increase the staff's understanding of older people with chronic health conditions, mental health disorders, and addiction disorders. This training may help to reduce stigma that is sometimes encountered by older adults in long-term care facilities (Lau-Ng et al., 2020). The unique concerns of women aging with HIV and the necessity to prepare for the future needs of older people living with HIV are discussed in more detail in Section IV.

Nationwide, Spence et al. (2022) emphasize the benefits of ongoing training and education for all healthcare providers, especially in obtaining sexual and drug use history and increasing knowledge about HIV prevention and transmission. Additionally, Lehman et al. (2014) determined 33 states still have HIV-specific criminal laws that require disclosure of HIV to sexual and needle-sharing partners. Most of these laws were enacted before the use of antiretroviral medications, which lower the risk of transmission. Furthermore, these laws often result in a high proportion of prosecutions for low-risk behavior and do not reduce the number of new transmissions (Lazzarini et al., 2013). To remedy this situation of ineffective and outdated laws, Lazzarini et al. (2013) and Lehman et al. (2014) recommend (1) reviewing and updating existing state laws, (2) writing prosecutorial guidelines to limit prosecutions, and (3) researching the impact of and cost of these criminalization laws. Lazzarini et al. (2013) further recommend promoting broad-based harm reduction public policy messages to reduce the number of new HIV transmissions and to increase the likelihood of HIV disclosure.

By educating family, friends, healthcare providers, employers, faith communities, and the public, HIV stigma will be reduced. Additionally, updating public policy and laws will create a society more accepting and supportive of people living with HIV. As people living with HIV become more accepted and visible in society, more people will feel comfortable disclosing their positive status to others. These disclosures will help to reduce HIV stigma through increased awareness of HIV.

Personal Connection

Challenging HIV Stigma with Education

As a lifelong learner and educator, I have witnessed the power of education to transform lives. After realizing I was living with HIV, I immediately sought to educate myself about how to live with HIV and about how HIV was affecting my body. I was also very concerned about what would happen if my employer discovered I was HIV-positive. As a public-school teacher, I feared my employer would dismiss me for being positive. Even though I knew I was legally protected under the Americans with Disabilities Act (U.S. Department of Justice, 2008), I also knew how easily an employer could obfuscate reasons for dismissal to hide discrimination resulting from being HIV-positive. Additionally, I feared the reactions of parents, students, other teachers, and community members if they realized I was HIV-positive. My fears increased when I decided to speak publicly about living with HIV. Each time I spoke, I had to remind myself of the importance of my message and the need to educate others. I knew I was helping to challenge HIV stigma each time I shared my story.

Over my career, I have taught in several school districts, and I have disclosed my positive status to some of my employers. However, most of my employers did not know. My main reason for nondisclosure was my fear of being stigmatized for living with HIV, even though I was fortunate to never face discrimination after disclosing. Another reason I did not disclose my positive status was that my position in some districts was temporary, such as a summer school or semester contract. This point generates another deliberation on the layers of disclosure in an organization. For instance, in a school district, I could disclose to the superintendent, the human resource supervisor, the school board, my building principal, the school nurse, my teaching colleagues, or to parents and students. Each of these audiences requires its own analysis of the consequences of disclosure. Another factor is the requirement to disclose to new people each time I change teaching positions. For example, if I moved to a new building, I would need to inform a new principal or colleagues. Also, as people retire or are replaced, I would need to inform their replacements of my positive status. A final reason for nondisclosure is that living with HIV has no impact on my ability to teach, and therefore, my positive status does not need to be disclosed to an employer.

While I was conducting my dissertation research, interview participants revealed their concerns about disclosing their positive status to others and about experiencing HIV stigma. They also recounted their efforts to educate others about HIV and how education helped them to live with HIV. Listening to participants' concerns renewed my desire to share my journey with others to help challenge HIV stigma in society. In this section, I will summarize some of the steps I took to educate myself and others while developing HIV endurance.

As I mentioned in the preface, when I first learned I was HIV-positive, I went to several bookstores and the library to get books about HIV. However, I did not find any books about HIV. This surprised me. I wondered why there weren't any books about HIV since it was 1998—over ten years since the first HIV cases were diagnosed. When I spoke to my HIV specialist, Susan, about this lack of books on HIV, she gave me several pamphlets and *POZ* magazines to read. Also, when I expressed my concern of my physical weakness and lack of appetite, she suggested I read the book *Nutrition and HIV: A New Model for Treatment* by Mary Romeyn, which had just been released in March 1998. This book gave me some good suggestions about foods I could eat to help rebuild my strength.

Susan also gave me a copy of the book *HIV Law: A Survival Guide to the Legal System for People Living with HIV* by Paul Hampton Crockett, which had been published in April 1997. This book opened my eyes to the unique legal considerations for people living with HIV. I appreciated the explanations, advice, and resources the author gave. By reading this book, I was connected to the AIDS Law Project of PA, which is based in Philadelphia. I made an appointment with the AIDS Law Project to have them help me write a living will and to designate a healthcare power of attorney. While I was there, I recognized the critical work the AIDS Law Project of PA was engaged in, and I committed myself to help fund their work in the future.

As my health improved, I continued to seek out and read more information about HIV. Susan made it easy for me to get HIV information by always having the latest *POZ* magazines easily accessible in her exam room. I also received pamphlets from Project Inform and got other books about living with HIV. When I started to speak publicly, I gave some of the information I was acquiring to others to educate them on how HIV affects a person's life. I also shared the information I learned about living with HIV with my family, friends, and sexual partners as I disclosed my HIV-positive status to them.

After meeting and speaking to Christine, as I recounted in the preface, I joined WORLD and started receiving their newsletter, which focused on women's experiences with HIV. I also started to attend conferences and to speak to other women who were living with HIV. My attendance at these conferences helped me to keep abreast of the latest scientific research on HIV. I also received inspiration from the advocacy work of other conference attendees.

Additionally, I went on some weekend HIV retreats. These retreats allowed me to listen to other people living with HIV and to learn about their lives. I was also able to share my concerns about living with HIV and get advice from other people who were also living with HIV. The intimacy and safe space created by the retreats' weekend seclusion encouraged us to share our life stories. By sharing our life stories, we were educating each other, increasing social capital, and empowering each other to share our stories with others. Through the act of sharing our stories with others, we humanized HIV, showing people that anyone can get HIV and that people shouldn't be stigmatized for having HIV.

Four Key Takeaways

HIV Stigma

- People living with HIV may experience stigma from their family, friends, sexual partners, healthcare providers, employers, and public.
- To protect themselves from stigma, people living with HIV practice strategic disclosures, where they disclose their status to selective others, and concealment, where they attempt to pass as HIV-negative.
- Education is a powerful means to reduce the stigma associated with HIV at the micro, meso, and macro levels of society.
- People living with HIV may also benefit from participating in a support group where they can discuss encounters with HIV stigma and brainstorm solutions with others.

SECTION III

HIV and Identity

Chapter 8

HIV's Effect on Identity

This section examines the effects of HIV on a woman's identity. Finding out you are living with HIV is very traumatic. A person needs to incorporate their positive status into their prior identity. In this chapter, I first offer my findings of the ways that living with HIV has affected the identities of my research participants. Then, I outline some of the methods the women employ to cope with living with HIV. These coping strategies include prayer, advocacy, education, and support groups. In chapter 9, I summarize some of the key research on how living with a chronic illness affects a person's identity and on how a person processes a traumatic event using the stages of posttraumatic growth. I also examine how people preserve self and incorporate chronic illness into their life story. In chapter 10, I use my journal entries from 1999 to 2002 to illustrate the path I took as I worked to integrate HIV into my identity and to resolve my spiritual beliefs and practices.

This chapter summarizes my findings of the effects of HIV on a woman's identity and how interview participants cope with living with HIV. At the end of my interviews, I asked each woman how she thought HIV had affected her life and her identity and how she copes with living with HIV. Here are some of their answers to these questions.

HOW HIV AFFECTS IDENTITY

When asked how HIV has affected her sense of identity, Ava asserted, "I'm not HIV! I have an illness. We have a chronic illness, and HIV does not make us. Take me on who I am, not what illness I carry 'cause HIV is not me." However, Ava did offer her understanding of HIV's effect on her current lifestyle and how living with HIV changed her life course: "I think it saved my life, basically, because I was on a self-destructive pattern of drugs and alcohol. I didn't care about the next person. I was a selfish person, and now, I'm more giving and loving and open; and I'm more in tune with my higher power than I've ever been. And I can contribute that to HIV or having being diagnosed; I'll put it that way. What else was it? I truly feel that I'm a better person."

Concurring with Ava's sentiment about how HIV affected her life, Kendra revealed how living with HIV has helped her to recover from her addiction to drugs: "It's made me more spiritual. It also has helped me to become clean and sober. HIV has saved my life."

Hailey offered words of encouragement to other positive women as she expressed her sense of identity: "You're a positive woman; you're a strong woman; you're a woman of character; and I know you're a woman of faith. This woman refused to be used, so crying at night, trying to figure out just who I am is now history. My life is now glistening. This is the real me!"

Nevaeh, when asked about how HIV has affected her life, shared the following reflection:

> For me, HIV, I was a very shy person believe it or not. Yeah, HIV for me has—I'm more outgoing. I have a sense of myself that I don't think I would've had if I had not gotten the virus. HIV has made me do my spiritual work but really to know who I am, to know who God has made me, so, for me—I know a lot of people would say, 'How can you say that HIV was good for you?'—HIV was good for me because I was doing some crazy things at sixteen, seventeen years old, and I think if I had not got HIV, I would probably be dead. HIV has taught me who I am. I have a very good sense of self-worth. I know who God has made me and created me to be; so, HIV has been good for me.

In contrast to the above statements, some interview participants felt HIV affected them in more negative ways. For example, Michelle revealed, "I'm more guarded now." After receiving her diagnosis, Destiny remembered, "I went from way up here to way down here." However, years later after speaking publicly about her HIV to a group of young women, Destiny remarked that they gave her a standing ovation while shouting, "She's a hope shot!" Destiny went on to concur with Nevaeh's viewpoint about the positive effect of HIV, sharing a conversation she had with some of her friends, "At this point, I said, 'You might not see it,'—'cause my friends were like, 'What did she say?'—I said, 'but there's a blessing in this.' They were like, 'How could you say there's a blessing in something like that?' 'Cause it totally changed my life. I'm more responsible to my health."

After receiving their diagnosis of HIV, the women began to employ a variety of coping strategies to incorporate HIV into their identities and to sustain their lives as they lived with HIV.

COPING WITH HIV

The women I interviewed offered several ways they cope with living with HIV and where they draw their strength from each day. These positive coping strategies involve prayer, advocacy, education, and support groups.

Prayer

Many of the women I interviewed expressed the importance of their faith and spiritual practices in helping them to manage the trauma of living with HIV each day. For example, when asked where she obtained her daily strength, Laila responded, "My relationship with God, I always been in church, all my life. I always, always had a spiritual connection with my God. Yes, but I think it was when—within the years after I found out that I was positive, where I was made a believer." Josie concurred, "I pray every morning." Nevaeh said, "My strength comes from God, no ifs, ands, or buts about it. My strength—the only way I'm this strong is because of God that lives inside of me. If I did not have Him and I didn't have my spiritual family and my spiritual background, I would be somewhere in a nuthouse. Honestly, I would."

Additionally, Tamara asserted, "So, I draw my strengths from—my first strength comes from an inter-spiritual belief. I'm spiritual. I have a Catholic background, and that's where my first strength comes from. My second strength comes from my family support. I have a family that supports and loves me regardless of my status."

As a part of their coping strategies, some women use music or art to connect spiritually. For instance, when asked where she draws her strength, Kendra said, "My main way is through music, through music and prayer, you know. Yeah, music, music, that's my way. Music and the word, the word is the truth. It puts me in tune with God. From spiritualities, spirituality because music is about spirituality." Moreover, Salena described how her art helped her: "They display all of my artwork at the convention. They had a little storyboard about how I am very artistic and about my HIV and how I use my talents to express my feelings and thoughts. I use my art as a way to express myself."

In addition, prayer and spiritual practices often help to sustain women in their advocacy work, which is discussed next.

Advocacy

Another positive coping strategy used by interview participants was to become advocates and speak publicly about HIV to educate others about HIV prevention. The women reported how they gained strength from their HIV prevention and volunteer work. For example, Destiny communicated how her advocacy work helps her cope:

> It helps me—well, for me to be the positive; first of all, before I even became an advocate, I used to pray to be positive. Well just give me something positive to say to somebody; and I'd had no idea—I even told people, I said, 'I don't know if people usually pray for stuff like that, but that was something I always prayed for. I always prayed to be positive. I wanna be able to say something positive to somebody when they in a bad place.' So, who knew He would take me here? But He knew; He built me, so He brought me here for this reason; like, you have something positive to say 'cause you asked for it; now, I gave it to you; now, you tell them because they are people come in here totally devastated. He has blessed me so many other kinda ways. He increased my positivity. He put me in a job that I wasn't looking for. I never, ever applied for this job.

Hailey concurred, saying, "God wants to use me right here, right now to be a witness to those, not just concerning the Bible but concerning health issues, because this thing is real. It's real, and I'm living with it. I'm a witness."

Ava shared that one of her coping strategies is helping others: "When I'm here at work, I truly try to help."

Josie's suggestion for other positive women was, "You have to advocate for yourself. Secrets hurt. Keeping something in is going to keep you from being healthy. A lot of people don't ask questions; don't know what questions to ask; and some doctors don't encourage it."

By asking questions, women expand their knowledge of HIV, educating themselves, and often educating others about HIV as shown next.

Education

Each woman spoke about the importance of educating herself and others about HIV. For instance, Tamara described herself as a "graduate of the Black AIDS Institute." Salena summarized her educational process: "This year, I graduate at TEACH Outside, regular TEACH, and they helped me so much with the whole depression and the postpartum depression and being happy with who I am as of right now." Laila remarked, "I went to detox. I steady kept going to the groups and support groups and everything and getting educated on it. It's important that you get educated, so you can educate other people."

The other participants were equally passionate about educating others about HIV prevention. Tamara expounded on her efforts to educate young people: "I'm always talking about safer sex. If they don't have the knowledge of transmission, I make sure I educate them." Specifically, while speaking to young women, Tamara emphasized the importance of "helping them make sure that they know all the information they need to know so that they don't put themselves at risk for HIV or any other sexually transmitted diseases. I make sure that I tell other women who are negative, if you are going to have multiple partners, here's what you need to do to protect yourself 'cause you really don't know anyone's status, like [unless] they go to the doctor's, and you get them tested."

Josie's HIV prevention and awareness work also involves "educating young people with a course, 'After You Know, What Do You Do?'—strictly about HIV awareness." She said that she "encourages everybody's grandchildren to go to their grandparents and tell my story and encourage their grandparents to get tested." Josie revealed her reason for educating others: "Looking at my own ignorance, I said there are a lot of people like me out there, and I realized nobody was talking to older people. Everybody needs to be tested."

To further reach out to the public and promote the message of HIV awareness, Ava explained, "We also have classes for those that are negative to teach about the virus, what goes on with the body, how we can live stronger, healthier, productive lives. So, learning about classes in their area or groups in their area that teaches education 'cause education has always been power in any form." Talking about her reasons for educating others, Ava continued, "I want them to know that there's people out here that love them regardless of whatever and that we just have an illness. So as long as I'm speaking on it, okay, I'm HIV-positive. Now what, anything else you had to say? I know my status. Do you know yours? Now, let's go get tested. Let's talk. Let's share."

From her years of public speaking and educating young people about HIV prevention, Irene concurred with Ava's statement. "Proper education is key because there's so many myths and misinformation out there even today, and things do change," Irene related. "And even as I'm out sharing my heart and doing educational programs, I implement not only the basic education, but I share parts of my story. I get both components in, and when I share the personal side, it's not out of sympathy but empathy. But many times, that is a component that people don't get a chance to hear about."

In closing our interview, Hailey's shout-out to other women was an attempt to inspire and educate other positive women:

> There is hope in your life. There is hope in whatever it is you desire to do with your life; being HIV-positive, you can accomplish it. I'm gonna accomplish my dreams. Reach out to your dreams, and most importantly, reach one and

teach one. Somebody needs to know right where you are. Somebody needs to get tested right in your atmosphere. Somebody needs to know their status right now. Don't be afraid; don't be ashamed to tell 'em where you are and what you're doing. Come forth ladies! It's time to stand up, so that we can help save our people.

The importance of women being together and educating each other about HIV is discussed next with an emphasis on the power of support groups to help women cope with living with HIV.

Support Groups

Interview participants spoke of the importance of a support system, which is usually enhanced by social media. Women's support systems usually consist of family, friends, and other positive women. For example, Salena shared, "So finally, I disclosed on Facebook, and everybody was like, 'Oh my goodness! I didn't know, and I'm here to support.' Every time I have a problem, I could post something on Facebook."

Laila revealed the importance of attending her support group meetings: "The groups that they had—they had a women's group every other Saturday of the month. It was just so wonder[ful]—and we would get so much information on Saturdays." Michelle explained that her support group attendance helped her to form lifelong friendships:

> We have group sessions; we talk about everything. We talk about addiction, and I mentioned that I was HIV-positive. And when I got really sick once, they came and checked on me; and when I had my hip surgery, they just took care of me. They brought dinners every day, yeah, yeah. They stayed my friends, and I still talk to them. And those were people that I met in the recovery process of the drug addiction. The ladies in my building, we all came through the same drug treatment. Now, we all have apartments in the same building; and they're just fine with it. Some of them'll call me and check on me.

Some women also became mentors to younger women, helping to guide them on their HIV journeys and offering encouragement to persevere. For instance, Tamara reported how she mentors younger women: "I'm twenty-one years positive, and by looking at me, you couldn't tell that, right? And I think it helps other people who are newly diagnosed to hear from women who've been living with it for a long time and see their journey—that their journey's a positive one; and their journey, as they move forward, will be a positive one as well."

In the next chapter, I summarize key research findings that bolster the evidence I presented in chapter 8. I discuss how chronic illness affects a person's identity and how an HIV diagnosis often acts as a traumatic event and ambiguous loss in a person's life. This is because a diagnosis of HIV causes a woman to revise her identity to incorporate her positive status and educate herself to preserve herself and cope with the posttraumatic stress of living with HIV.

Chapter 9

Incorporating HIV into One's Identity

Becoming infected with HIV is like an ambiguous loss because a woman loses parts of her old identity as a seronegative person (D'Amore, 2019). According to Boss (2007), an ambiguous loss is an unclear loss that creates uncertainty. An ambiguous loss impacts a woman and her loved ones because of the lack of information and closure stemming from the loss (Boss, 2007). There is a lack of meaning in the situation, which results in complicated grief (Boss, 2007). This chapter examines how a diagnosis of HIV prompts a reshaping of identity and how it affects identity roles, especially for women.

CHRONIC ILLNESS AND TIME

According to Bury (1982; 1991), a chronic illness causes a biographical disruption, impacting a person's self-concept and relationship with others. Chronic illness affects a person's identity and self-concept, bringing consequences for a person in terms of symptoms and the different meanings associated with a chronic illness at different stages of life (Charmaz, 1991). Because the body and self are connected, a person living with chronic illness needs to reevaluate former views of self and prior assumptions to reconstruct the self and incorporate new experiences, knowledge, and meanings (Charmaz, 2002).

For this reason, being diagnosed with a chronic illness is viewed as a traumatic event because of the initial shock of diagnosis and the need to incorporate the chronic illness into identity. However, as a person lives with a chronic illness, her experiences change in relation to time (Charmaz, 1991). Initially, a person may seek to understand and resolve past events, living in the past, and trying to determine how past events led to the present condition (Charmaz, 1991). When the present is insecure and unacceptable, a person may revisit the familiar past to find comfort and understanding. Charmaz (1991) found that a chronically ill person may remember idealized versions of self where she was healthy in a reconstructed past.

A chronic illness may also affect how a person lives in the present. For instance, chronically ill people often find themselves living in the here and now. According to Charmaz (1991), a person who is living with a chronic illness often does not want to miss a moment in life. She may try to live her life to the fullest by having a filled or intense present life, which is lived with passion and authenticity (Charmaz, 1991). At other times, chronically ill people may live in a present that is more relaxed, where they appreciate and enjoy each moment and are more emotionally engaged in relationships (Charmaz, 1991).

Chronic illnesses may also alter how people view their future. For example, people living with a chronic illness often tie their self-concept to future dreams and possibilities (Charmaz, 1991). If a person can recover from an illness or not have serious effects from the chronic illness, she may view her life with new possibilities and opportunities to make an ideal self (Charmaz, 1991). Furthermore, a person may envision an improved future, where she is able to plan for and hope for a more complete and fully realized self (Charmaz, 1991). However, when a person envisions a hopeless future, filled with fear and dependency, she may feel trapped and may suffer negative emotions, such as anger, depression, and self-pity, Charmaz observes (1991). When people living with a chronic illness situate their present life in the future, projecting their current self-concept into the future, a taken-for-granted future is created because the present provides a path to the future (Charmaz, 1991). If the future does not work out as planned, then a person may become disillusioned. Lastly, in an everlasting future, a chronically ill person feels death is imminent, so she seeks to create an immortal self through religion, work, or other products, according to Charmaz (1991).

A diagnosis of a chronic illness often becomes the focal point of a person's life and, according to Charmaz (2008), prompts a transformation. This transformation helps people to manage their illness and find meaning in the illness experience. People living with chronic illnesses describe their experiences of transcendence and transformation in a similar manner as people who lived through a traumatic event (Charmaz, 2008). Additionally, Charmaz (2008) also reports that chronically ill people state they are more grateful, try to live more in the present, and often reorganize their priorities after being diagnosed with a chronic illness. Part of the transcendence means they view their bodies and their lives differently, aspiring to live with passion and purpose after surviving the turbulence of a chronic illness and gathering resiliency for the future (Charmaz, 2008).

The next section examines how living with the chronic illness of HIV affects women's identities.

IDENTITY HIERARCHY

Because a woman engages in a variety of societal roles, the disruption to identity caused by a diagnosis of HIV generates a reshaping of other societal fronts. According to Tsarenko and Polonsky (2011), the presence of HIV acts to amplify the process of interruption in identity change, while adding a layer of complexity related to interrelationship between a category-based (HIV-positive) identity and a role-based (parent, employee, etc.) identity. This amplification is cyclical, requiring a person to engage in self-acceptance and ownership throughout life (Tsarenko & Polonsky, 2011).

Additionally, there is a hierarchy of identities that chronically ill people move through to find meaning and to live with their illness (Charmaz, 1983, 1991, 1994; Nixon & Renwick, 2003). In ascending order, these four preferred identities are: the Salvaged Self, the Contingent Personal Identity, the Restored Self, and the Supernormal Social Identity (Charmaz, 1994; Nixon & Renwick, 2003). As women reshape their societal fronts to incorporate the disruption to identity caused by HIV, they attempt to reestablish their self-concept (Ciambrone, 2003; Goffman, 1959). At first, most women internalize the shame and stigma associated with HIV (Ciambrone, 2003). The experience of shame may reinforce self-perceptions of damage and weakness, causing some women, especially women who previously encountered abuse or trauma, to engage in more avoidant, negative, and submissive behaviors (Ciambrone, 2003; Persons et al., 2010). Furthermore, Ciambrone (2003) determined other women may initially withdraw from society, feeling hopeless and depressed, but then, reorganize to make new sense of their lives and preserve their identity as discussed next.

Preserving Self

Stets and Burke (2000) determined identities are organized in a hierarchy with the most activated identity at the top and less activated identities appearing based on a situation. Moreover, the self is influenced by society, and the self also influences society (Stets & Burke, 2000). People act to keep perceptions of themselves in situations, taking actions to modify situations so self-perception is consistent despite situational disturbances (Stets & Burke, 2000). At the micro level, a person feels most authentic when her identity is verified. For example, a woman's identity is verified when she enacts certain roles in her associated groups, develops inter- and intragroup relations at the meso-level, or commits to a role to support her associated group at the macro level of society (Stets & Burke, 2000).

The theory of how people preserve self while living with a chronic illness involves five interrelated stages. According to Vann-Ward et al. (2017), the first stage of preserving self involves making sense of symptoms and acting on these symptoms. When people first receive a diagnosis, they often react with emotions ranging from shock to relief because they finally have an answer to the cause of their symptoms (Vann-Ward et al., 2017). The second stage is how a diagnosis is often a defining turning point because it causes an identity change and is a life-altering event (Vann-Ward et al., 2017). During this stage, individuals often seek information about their illness, join support groups, decide who to disclose to, and begin to accept their diagnosis (Vann-Ward et al., 2017). The third stage of preserving self, according to Vann-Ward et al. (2017), involves an identity dilemma, where individuals attempt to resolve reminders of their pre-illness identity with their new chronically ill identity. During this stage, individuals often feel disconnected, depressed, vulnerable, and isolated, according to Vann-Ward et al. (2017). As individuals work to establish new boundaries based on their chronic illness, they also develop new vigilance and protective actions according to the requirements of their chronic illness (Vann-Ward et al., 2017).

In the fourth stage of preserving self, individuals self-evaluate their abilities and plans, grieve their past self, sort out former activities that are no longer feasible, and adopt new activities (Vann-Ward et al., 2017). These new activities help to form new identities, which consist of three main types: 1) resentful, where people express blame and anger, 2) resolute, where people work to maintain their identities and fulfill prior responsibilities, and 3) reformulated, where people redefine themselves as living with a chronic illness and accept the reality of their diagnosis (Vann-Ward et al., 2017). During the final stage of preserving self, individuals balance risks and rewards by envisioning a future and accepting the conditions of their chronic illness. In this last stage, individuals often simplify their lives and try to maintain their independence by fulfilling their responsibilities and finding ways to serve others (Tedeschi et al., 1998; Vann-Ward et al., 2017). Figure 9.1 summarizes the main stages of preserving self after an identity disruption caused by a chronic illness diagnosis.

According to Vann-Ward et al. (2017), there are several strategies a person can employ to cope with living with a chronic illness and to preserve self. One main strategy for preserving self is to develop and maintain relationships with family members, healthcare providers, and employers to reinforce new identities and to maintain normalcy (Vann-Ward et al., 2017). A second strategy, according to Vann-Ward et al. (2017), involves taking actions to maintain former self and social identities while experiencing an identity dilemma.

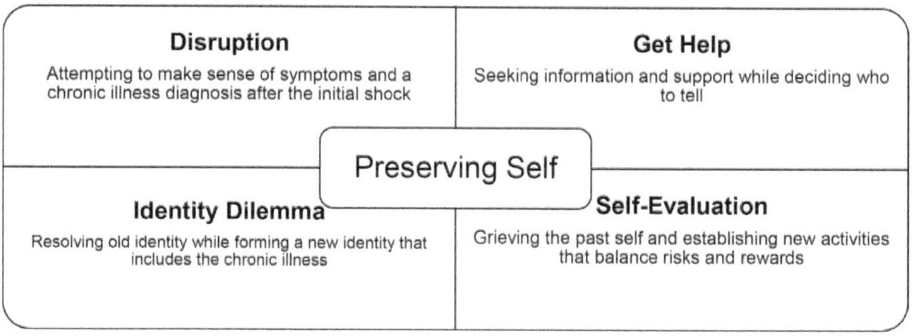

Figure 9.1. Components of Preserving Self (Data from Vann-Ward et al., 2017, figure created by author.)

Another strategy that helps to preserve self is to participate in mutual support groups to cope with chronic conditions and to make positive changes (Tedeschi et al., 1998; Vann-Ward et al., 2017). A fourth strategy to preserve self, according to Vann-Ward et al. (2017), is to participate in psychotherapy and counseling. Additionally, Tedeschi and Calhoun (1995) concluded that people often benefited from serving others, using humor, setting goals, and accepting traumatic events as opportunities for growth.

GROWTH AFTER TRAUMA

According to Tedeschi and Calhoun (1995), to make a traumatic event comprehensible, manageable, and meaningful, a person engages in a process of rumination, where she thinks often of the event and searches for meaning and goals resulting from the event. During rumination, a person experiences denial, acceptance, disengagement, and engagement, which challenge her schema and sense of the world (Tedeschi & Calhoun, 1995).

Several principles of personal growth help to make sense of a traumatic event, according to Tedeschi and Calhoun (1995). First, a person's schema needs to change after the traumatic event, which usually speeds up the development of a new schema because of the shock and distress caused by the trauma. A second principle is that certain assumptions, such as religious beliefs, are resistant to change and reduce the possibility of schema change and growth (Tedeschi & Calhoun, 1995). If a positive evaluation of the trauma is possible, a third principle is that growth will occur. However, different types of traumatic events will produce different types of growth, and personality characteristics also impact the possibility of growth, according to Tedeschi and Calhoun (1995). Another principle is that growth occurs when the trauma assumes the central part of a person's life story and that wisdom is the product of this growth (Tedeschi & Calhoun, 1995; Tedeschi et al., 1998). To grow after a traumatic event, a person needs to rewrite her life story and incorporate the traumatic event into her life.

The next section offers various coping methods that people employ to incorporate traumatic events into their lives.

COPING METHODS

Because becoming HIV-positive is a life-changing, traumatic event, a person's initial response is to manage the distress caused by the newly acquired positive status. Each person's prior orienting system of coping resources impacts the ability to cope with each new life event (Pargament, 1997). This orienting system also includes a person's commitments and beliefs. According to Pargament (1997), there are four methods people employ to seek significance through coping. The first method is *preservation,* where people try to preserve their lives and behaviors which existed before a tragic event (Pargament, 1997). The second method is *reconstruction,* where people obtain new skills, resources, and beliefs to obtain significance (Pargament, 1997). A third coping method, which is especially used in life-threatening situations, is a *revaluation of goals,* where a person's goals are reprioritized, redefining significance (Pargament, 1997). If the life event is severe or if the other three methods have not resulted in significance, then a person often *recreates their pathway and destination of significance*. People will change their habits, way of life, and goals in life, to find significance in new ways (Pargament, 1997).

People may also practice religious coping, which includes some positive aspects, such as expressing spirituality, believing there is meaning in life, and connecting with others (Pargament, 1997). There are also some negative aspects associated with religious coping, such as struggling with religion and the concept of God, believing the devil influences life events, and reappraising religious faith and significance (Pargament, 1997).

In the next section, I will discuss the opportunity and process for posttraumatic growth, which includes the component of spirituality.

POSTTRAUMATIC GROWTH

After a traumatic event, a person moves along parallel paths of spiritual emergency and spiritual emergence (Bray, 2010; Grof & Grof, 1990; Tedeschi & Calhoun, 1995; Tedeschi et al., 1998). A spiritual emergency occurs when a person confronts a crisis, suffers inner distress, and reevaluates prior beliefs

(Bray, 2010; Grof & Grof, 1990; Tedeschi & Calhoun, 1995; Tedeschi et al., 1998). Spiritual emergence involves integrating new knowledge into a prior narrative (Bray, 2010; Grof & Grof, 1990; Tedeschi & Calhoun, 1995; Tedeschi et al., 1998). Both paths involve rumination and awareness of conscious and unconscious material through self-disclosure using prayer, writing, talking, creative expression, or physical activity (Bray, 2010; Grof & Grof, 1990; Tedeschi & Calhoun, 1995; Tedeschi et al., 1998). Additionally, there is often an extensive period of narrative development and schema change after a traumatic event because a person is processing and remaking meaning in her life (Bray, 2010; Grof & Grof, 1990; Tedeschi & Calhoun, 1995; Tedeschi et al., 1998). A person will go through a continuum of distress with impeded and unimpeded processing depending on the amount of posttraumatic growth, narrative wisdom, and improved functioning a person has (Bray, 2010; Grof & Grof, 1990; Tedeschi & Calhoun, 1995; Tedeschi et al., 1998).

According to Gilbert and Wright (2003), transformation implies a new attitude and behavior, where a woman may leave abusive relationships, reconcile with family members, maintain her sobriety, reconnect spiritually, and realize she has the right to determine her reaction to the conditions of her life. As discussed earlier, women often use their HIV diagnosis to reevaluate their lives, to change their circumstances, and to reignite their hope, optimism, and spiritual connections to empower themselves to improve their life circumstances (Gilbert & Wright, 2003). To preserve their identities, women often employ active coping strategies, like those previously discussed in chapter 8. These activities increase self-awareness and acceptance by highlighting the positive aspects of living with HIV (Ciambrone, 2003; D'Amore, 2019). Additionally, by educating others and engaging in advocacy, women reflect their ability to transcend a negative self-image of living with HIV to emphasize a life of acceptance, generosity, and helpfulness (Ciambrone, 2003; D'Amore, 2019).

REWRITING A LIFE STORY

After a traumatic event and much effort coping with the event, a person can often incorporate the traumatic event into her life story, find new meaning in life, and change her philosophy of life, which may include a spiritual component, according to Tedeschi and Calhoun (1995). People use four different narratives to respond to illness and redraw their life maps (Frank, 1995). Over the course of an illness, these narratives are communicated repeatedly and interchangeably (Frank, 1995). The restitution narrative, according to Frank (1995), is characterized by a contrast between life before and life after successful treatment, with a goal of restoring a person's concept of her healthy self. The chaos narrative is characterized by a lack of voice because the individual encounters a lack of control of her disease and medicine's inability to control the disease (Frank, 1995).

In contrast, a quest narrative restores a person's voice by framing illness as a journey, where the person accepts her illness and becomes a proactive narrative agent (Frank, 1995). Quest narratives are based on recollection, solidarity, and inspiration, where the past is recollected and accepted, and the storyteller uses her voice to witness with other sufferers according to Frank (1995). By becoming a witness to disease and suffering, a person moves from a quest narrative to a testimony to contribute to the social construction of the illness, taking it out of the private body world and into the social world (Frank, 1995). Stories are embedded in contexts and often signify a transformation of self that emerges through suffering and struggling to preserve self (Charmaz, 2009).

In the next chapter, I apply the concepts of preserving self and posttraumatic growth to my life as a woman living with HIV.

Chapter 10

My HIV Testimony

In this chapter, I analyze how I used rumination and a restitution narrative to preserve myself and to incorporate HIV into my identity. This chapter draws on some of my journal entries from 1999 to 2002.

RUMINATION

During the first months after receiving my HIV diagnosis, I spent many evenings and weekends reading about HIV and AIDS. I read about people who were living with HIV and about people who died of AIDS. My main support person during this time was a male friend who I initially disclosed my positive status to and Susan, my HIV specialist. My other sources of comfort and support were the various helplines and hotlines that existed at that time. I was able to call these telephone numbers and speak to others who were familiar with managing antiretroviral medications and the feelings associated with living with HIV. My coping strategy was to read everything I could find about HIV and AIDS and then to think about and ruminate about how my life was before HIV and how I wanted to live my life with HIV. I spent hours journaling and ruminating about my life, my choices, and the consequences of my choices.

When I discovered I was positive, I saw it as a death sentence. My health had already started to suffer from HIV, and I had a lot of respect for the power of the virus to destroy my body's immune system. I acknowledged I could die at any time, and I wanted to prepare for death. Because I was Catholic, I decided my first step to prepare for my death was to speak to a priest about becoming HIV-positive. The priest I met with listened to me as I cried and recounted how I became positive. I announced to the priest that I wanted to prepare myself to die, and I asked for his advice. The priest suggested I return to the church and begin to attend weekly Mass. At that point in my life, I attended church periodically but not every week. I thanked the priest for his time, but I knew I needed to do more spiritual work before I would be at peace.

I continued to ruminate and write in my journal. Then, in January 2000, I went to my first HIV retreat. After I spoke to the priest at this retreat about all my guilt for becoming infected with HIV and my belief that I was going to die soon, he advised, "You are still trying to be a good little Catholic girl, and you need to grow up and become a Christian woman." He also suggested, "You have to understand your faith in a way that you are comfortable with your beliefs." After he recommended this, I realized being a Christian woman means being more Christlike. For me, being Christlike means acting from a place of unconditional love and promoting peace in the world. This insight led me to conclude this is the work I need to do in the world.

I continued to write in my journal trying to process my positive status and my religious beliefs. Multiple journal entries describe my gratefulness for having the opportunity to take the lifesaving antiretrovirals, my guilt associated with other people dying of AIDS, and my struggle with speaking publicly as a woman living with HIV. For example, in January 2002, I wrote:

> I am very happy to be alive. I know my time is limited. In Africa, two million people die every year of AIDS! I am so fortunate to have the privilege to take medications. I really need to make the most of the time I am given and to positively impact as many lives as possible. I know without the antiretrovirals, I would have been dead two years ago. I'll be lucky to live for another ten years. Ten thousand people die every day of AIDS around the world! I feel like the walls are closing in. I need to continue to speak publicly about HIV to try to prevent people from becoming positive. I pray to God that I will be given the inner strength and backbone I need to stand tall and proud. I pray I will speak loud and clear. I pray I will remain positive even in the face of ridicule. I pray my message saves the lives of others and contributes to making the world a better place.

I also spent a lot of my first couple of years of journaling reminiscing about my childhood, teen, and college years. These memories helped me to center myself and make sense of my pre-HIV life. Slowly, I was incorporating my pre-HIV self with myself as a woman living with HIV.

PRESERVING MYSELF

During the first nine months after receiving my HIV diagnosis, I made sense of my symptoms and used my HIV diagnosis as a turning point, which altered my life plans. To help me during the first two stages of preserving self, I relied on my relationships with my family, friends, and HIV specialist. I then moved into the third and fourth stages of preserving self. My identity dilemma was most evident each time I spoke publicly about HIV prevention. Each time I spoke publicly I had to balance my old identity with my new identity as a woman living with HIV. I also began to grieve my past self, evaluate my abilities and plans, and adopt new activities to envision a new future. During this time, I worked to accept my new identity as a woman living with HIV, to simplify my life, to maintain my independence, and to find new ways to serve others.

To accomplish these stages of preserving self, I attended occasional HIV retreats, accepted my HIV diagnosis as an opportunity for growth, and formed a friendship with Christine, who offered me a model of a woman living with HIV. Because of the supportive people I had early in my HIV diagnosis and my attendance at HIV retreats, I was able to incorporate my HIV-positive status into my pre-HIV identity. This new identity allowed me to speak publicly about being a woman living with HIV to try to influence the views of other people in society about positive women.

MOVING TOWARDS TESTIMONY

In April 1999, my HIV specialist, Susan, asked me to speak with her at an upcoming presentation on women and HIV. At first, I declined her request, believing I could never share my positive status with others. However, Susan convinced me that I could show people that HIV doesn't discriminate and that anyone can become infected with HIV. She argued that I didn't fit the stereotype that people have when they think about a woman who is living with HIV. Also, I realized by speaking publicly, I could help to educate others about HIV and help to reduce the stigma surrounding HIV. Therefore, less than a year after my diagnosis, I started speaking publicly to educate others about HIV prevention. I even spoke publicly before disclosing my positive status to my family members.

However, each time I spoke publicly, I wrestled with the consequences of speaking publicly and living publicly as a positive woman. For example, my journal entry from June 2000 states, "Each step I take towards being more public gets a little scarier. I'm scared of the consequences when people find out. I'm scared of losing my job, my apartment, and my benefits. I'm scared of losing my friends and family. I'm scared of dying and not having resolved my religious beliefs." As I moved from a restitution narrative to a quest and testimonial narrative, I continued to work to preserve my pre-HIV self while incorporating my new identity as a woman living with HIV. This process of preserving self was enhanced by the spiritual development work I became involved with in October 2001.

MY SPIRITUAL JOURNEY

When I started attending the spiritual development group, I was finally able to resolve my dilemma around my religious beliefs. The spiritual development group had emerged from a grief support group for people who had suffered the death of a family member. I attended the spiritual development group twice a month on Wednesdays evenings for several years. We met in a church meeting room, but it was nondenominational. These workshops provided the answers I was looking for because the sessions addressed the concerns I had as I prepared to die. I was introduced to the following spiritual principles: (1) Be Here Now; (2) Kindness Towards Self, Loved Ones, Neutral People, and Enemies; (3) Developing the Attitude of Gratitude; (4) Developing Patience; (5) Acceptance of Self, Others, and What Is; (6) Developing Compassion; (7) Developing the Attitude of Forgiveness; and (8) Developing the Attitude of Love (Dunnavent, 2003; D'Amore, 2021). Additionally, I learned about the attitudinal pillars of mindfulness, which include non-judging, patience, beginner's mind, trust, non-striving, acceptance, and letting go (Dunnavent, 2003; D'Amore, 2021).

I then started to apply these spiritual principles and attitudinal pillars of mindfulness to improve my mindset and life. I was able to resolve the guilt I felt about getting infected with HIV. I was also able to forgive myself and my partner. This journal entry from September 2002 illustrates my efforts to practice forgiveness and acceptance:

> I forgive myself for not listening to my inner voice that warned me not to get involved with the man who infected me with HIV. I also forgive the man who infected me with HIV. Now, I'm going to start living even more fully than before. Life is too precious to waste a single moment. I want to live more truthfully and truer to myself. I lost my way and my beliefs, but now, I am healing. I will be stronger because of all this, and I will appreciate everything on a new level. Living with HIV is an ongoing lesson in humility, shame, pride, fear, joy, anger, scariness, bravery, weakness, strength, compassion, distrust, responsibility, forgiveness, and discrimination. I have all these feelings at different times. I believe when you are living with HIV, these emotions are exaggerated in size and frequency.

The most important benefit from my spiritual development groupwork was that I was able to resolve my relationship with the Catholic church and find a way to be comfortable with my practice of the Catholic faith. I built a toolkit of useful spiritual practices that I can employ throughout my daily life and that help me to feel ready to die in a peaceful manner when that time comes.

Personal Connection

My Spiritual Toolkit

In appendix C, I offer a summary of the eight spiritual principles and the corresponding attitudinal pillars of mindfulness. In this section, I give a brief overview of how I use these spiritual principles and attitudinal pillars of mindfulness in my daily life and how their use has helped me to sustain my HIV endurance.

Shortly after learning I was HIV-positive in 1998, I read that AIDS could be understood as the "Accelerated Inner Discovery of Self." This expression impressed on me that becoming HIV-positive often acts as a catalyst to prepare for death. As I mentioned in the preface, I spent a lot of time reading the essays in the book *From a Burning House: The AIDS Project Los Angeles Workshop Collection*, which was published in June 1996. From the essays, I saw how the men were using journaling to reflect on their lives as they prepared to die of AIDS. Their words helped me to understand the benefits of journaling and reflection when living with a chronic illness.

In 2000, each time my friend Christine and I would speak to each other, she would elaborate on the benefits of the spiritual development group she was attending. Christine would encourage me to join, but I responded I wasn't ready to do the spiritual work involved. From the couple of HIV retreats I had attended, I recognized I had a great deal of spiritual work to do. Then, in 2001, I met Christine for dinner one night. She shared that the spiritual development group was starting an introductory course that was meeting just six times during the year to introduce people to the concepts of spiritual development. Given the limited time commitment required of the introductory course, I agreed to try it. After the introductory course ended, I decided to commit myself to the spiritual development process. I continued to join the spiritual development sessions until the group disbanded in 2010. Joining the spiritual development group helped me to identify and establish the core spiritual practices I now use every day as discussed next.

The first principle I learned was to be here now, which means to focus on and live in the present moment. In practice, this involves making eye contact with a speaker and listening with attention. It also involves seeing each moment with a beginner's mind, as a new opportunity to be fully present in whatever task I am engaged in. The second set of principles I acquired was to act with kindness towards myself, loved ones, neutral persons, and enemies. Demonstrating kindness in the world requires me to act with service to others and with nonjudgment. By serving others and not judging them, I can be a mirror of love to others, and my loving kindness may help to generate more kindness in the world.

My next spiritual principle was to develop the attitude of gratitude and to be thankful for all the blessings I have in my life each day. The spiritual principle of developing patience has been my focus for many years because it involves the mindfulness attitudinal pillars of tolerance and patience. In practice, I remind myself to be patient and to practice wait time throughout the day whenever I feel myself becoming impatient. By developing patience, I also help myself practice the other spiritual principles of being in the now, showing kindness to others, and being grateful.

The next set of spiritual principles are the practice of acceptance of self, others, and what is. By accepting myself, others, and what is, I act with non-judgment, acceptance, and non-striving. This means I accept myself, other people, and various situations as they currently are and then act with kindness, compassion, and forgiveness to bring more love into the world. The spiritual principle of developing compassion focuses on caring about others and acting with nonjudgment and empathy.

Developing the attitude of forgiveness involves the attitudinal pillar of mindfulness of letting go of past regrets and grievances. In practice, forgiveness means living in the present and forgiving past actions. The last spiritual principle is developing the attitude of love, which involves the attitudinal mindfulness pillar of trust. In practice, loving myself and others consists of trusting and forgiving other people while building relationships. All the spiritual principles are an ongoing practice, and the development of love, compassion, forgiveness, patience, acceptance, and gratitude require a lifetime of effort. These principles are best developed in relationship to other people. By practicing them, I strengthen my spiritual fortitude, and I help to foster the world's spiritual well-being.

Four Key Takeaways

HIV and Identity

- Living with a chronic illness affects a person's identity.
- To cope with living with HIV, women often engage in spiritual practices, join support groups, and participate in advocacy work.
- To preserve self, a person needs to integrate their chronic illness into their identity.
- Education helps people to cope with their chronic illness.

SECTION IV

HIV and Aging

Chapter 11

Experiences of Aging with HIV

In 2019, there were an estimated 1.2 million people living with HIV in the United States, and 263,900 of these positive people were women (CDC, 2022a). Additionally, there were 36,801 new HIV diagnoses in the United States in 2019, and of these new diagnoses, 6,999 were in women (CDC, 2022a). Out of these 6,999 women, 1,156 were aged 55 and older, accounting for 17% of the total number of women diagnosed with HIV in 2019 (CDC, 2022b). Furthermore, according to the National Institutes of Health (NIH, 2021), over half of the people living with HIV in the United States in 2018 were over the age of 50. Additionally, the number of people aging with HIV is increasing due to the effective antiretroviral therapies available and the increased efforts to diagnose and treat people who are at risk of HIV (NIH, 2021).

However, the topic of aging with HIV has not been extensively researched or developed because people living with HIV have only recently, since the widespread use of antiretrovirals, been able to enjoy a normal lifespan. During my interviews, several participants expressed their concerns of aging with HIV, especially finding supportive and knowledgeable healthcare providers who understand both the obstacles of living with HIV and aging. My participants also shared how aging with HIV helped them to find their purpose in life. In chapter 11, I share some of their personal experiences aging with HIV. Then, in chapter 12, I present a literature review on the topic of aging with HIV. In chapter 13, I offer some strategies society can implement to ease the aging journey for women living with HIV.

Some of the women I interviewed had experiences of aging with HIV that they mentioned during their interviews, even though I did not ask them directly about aging with HIV. Out of the seventeen women I interviewed, twelve of them were over the age of 50. Seven of the women were in the age range of 50 to 59, and five of the women were 60 to 69 years old. The women spoke about how aging with HIV has caused them to find and renew their life purposes. They also spoke about the importance of supportive HIV specialists, case managers, and support groups who are knowledgeable about the effects of aging with HIV and who can help women negotiate unexpected obstacles. Interview participants also expressed concerns about managing and treating their various health conditions, which were compounded by having HIV. Here are some examples of the responses the women shared with me.

FINDING PURPOSE

The main way the women found purpose in their lives was through service to other people. This service was often to family members and took the form of acting as a care provider and helping to educate the next generation. Other women spoke about their HIV advocacy work and their efforts to help educate others about HIV prevention.

For instance, Jada credited HIV for reuniting her family and renewing her sense of purpose as a mother and grandmother. She revealed how her relationship with her family strengthened after they helped her move out of the care of a nursing home. Jada, an African American woman in her late sixties, had stayed in a nursing home for four months in 1997. While she was there, she discovered she had almost died of AIDS. After learning of her HIV diagnosis, Jada called her husband, even though they had separated twenty years before. When her husband realized Jada was living with HIV, he stopped using drugs and started helping her transition out of the nursing home. Several years later, Jada's adult son and daughter forgave and accepted their father again after seeing how supportive he was of Jada. After resuming her work as a housekeeper, Jada continued to work until she retired at age 63. She affirmed that the closeness of her family has rejuvenated her spirit and given her a renewed purpose in life. Jada further asserted that her relationships with her husband, children, and grandchildren sustain her as she ages with HIV.

As an African American woman at the age of 54, Tamara credits her HIV for improving her health and renewing her purpose to live a healthy life. Tamara responded:

> Before I became positive, I was a working single mother. Life was good, but I can say that once I found out my status, it made me take care of myself more and see my doctor more often. For a lot of people who are positive, we tend to see the doctor more often than those who are negative; and we actually are healthier because we do that. So, I had a positive outlook once I found out, as I look back on it. I'm more connected to who I am. I'm more connected to taking care of myself and holistically and physically, and seeing my providers and taking my medications like I'm supposed to, and getting rest, and all the other things that comes into a good healthcare setting for a person who's positive.

At age 62, Esther, who identified as a single African American woman, spends her time volunteering for an AIDS Service Organization and helping other people cope with living with HIV. Esther reported how her volunteer work helped her find purpose in her life as she ages with HIV. Quiet, reserved, and private, Esther shared that she loves volunteering because she can help others and that she "lives in the now" while practicing her renewed faith.

Likewise, Josie said that her work as a peer advocate and public speaker allows her to build on her faith foundation, which focuses on serving others and living with purpose. At age 68, Josie was very open about her experiences living with HIV. She explained that her faith sustains her throughout her advocacy work educating others about HIV prevention.

Some of the women reported how aging with HIV renewed their purpose in living a spiritual life. For instance, Kendra credited HIV with helping to renew her relationship with God and her spiritual practices. She said that she finds peace through listening to religious music and daily prayers. Revealing the importance of her spiritual life, Kendra shared:

> Because of my connection with God, my spirituality has developed 'cause before, I was in my religion, but now, I have spirituality. I'm not talking about my physical life; I'm talking about my spiritual life because I'm trying to go to heaven, okay? So yes, HIV put me in tune with God. I mean, my God, not just people saying God, but my relationship has been birthed, and it's growing, and I'm grateful. I'm so grateful. I mean it's odd to say that, but that's where I am. Some people say, 'Oh, that's crazy!' But it's not for me 'cause I know where I'm heading and what my goal is in life. I wouldn't have been in touch with God without HIV in my life. I would've kept on with my merry, old life using drugs. Now, I'm on methadone, five milligrams. I guess it helped me to become clean and sober. I'm coming off methadone, but you know what I'm saying. I may have been still out there trying to use drugs and been dead or locked up again, or something like that—arrested again, without HIV changing my life and helping me to become clean and sober.

In addition to finding a renewed sense of purpose in life from aging with HIV, interview participants spoke about the importance of having supportive others in their lives who understood the complexities of aging with HIV, as discussed in the next section.

SUPPORTIVE AND KNOWLEDGEABLE CARE

The importance of knowledgeable healthcare providers and case managers was emphasized by several interview participants. Most of the time, they are satisfied with the care they are receiving from their HIV specialist, but they want that person to be more aware of the effects of aging. This sentiment was most clearly articulated by Josie, who mentioned her encounter with her supportive case manager: "I said, 'You know, I need either an Infectious Disease doctor or a Geriatric Specialist. I need someone that understands my problem of aging and my status; and this doctor, though she's a very good doctor, I don't think she has enough knowledge; she doesn't know as much as I do about me.' And so, I was assigned, like I said, the head of the department." Josie went on to clarify the benefits of a supportive case manager: "I do have a case manager person. And it was awesome because if I had an issue, I could call that case manager and say, 'I don't know what to do. I got this in the mail. I don't even understand what it's saying.' And she'd say, 'Bring it to me.' I'm here at least every couple weeks and drop it off for her."

Kendra, who is 52 and in recovery from drug addiction, talked about the importance of having a medical doctor who understands her and takes time to treat her needs:

> My HIV doctor is a good doctor! Oh God, I love my doctor! I had him at one clinic, and then, I followed him to another clinic. He doesn't rush me. He listens to me. He addresses my concerns. He gives me the information that I need. He doesn't agree with everything I say that I want, and he gives me the rationales why and makes me understand. He takes the time; he's a care provider—what a care provider's standards should be, plus some. He calls me at home; he checks on me. Yeah, my doctor calls me, if he's sent a prescription in, and he knows that previously I may have had a concern about getting a prescription. He did that last month; he did it a few months before; he's done it consistently in the past two years.

At age 62, Michelle echoed the importance of a medical care facility that includes services to treat HIV and other medical conditions:

> I have wonderful medical care! Any complaints that you have, they will get on it, either change your regiment, or give you a suggestion. My doctor told me that I should try tai chi because it's a movement thing and with the fibromyalgia, it's the joint stiffness—and they have a tai chi class on Saturday mornings. So, they do that, and it's a few other places that have the tai chi, and it's just to keep your range of motions, to keep you from being so stiff. But of course, the weather is what keeps them from going 'cause they're outside, and I can't be outside in the heat. During the summer, I can't do that tai chi outside.

In addition to fibromyalgia, Michelle described other medical conditions she lives with as she ages with HIV:

> Especially for me, the pain and stuff, then, I have so many medical conditions that cropped up from this—fibromyalgia; I have my hips, and I had the diabetic

> nerve pain; my hands swell, especially in the heat. My hands get puffy and fat, and the heat makes me absolutely dizzy. I will actually pass out, so I try to stay out of hot weather. I'm usually inside of an air-conditioned apartment, my apartment. So, I spent a lot of time home, but it's safer. I don't wanna pass out in the street—number one, embarrassment is too great for me—plus, I don't think people will respond to you; they'll think you're a drunk laying on the street, and I don't want that to happen to me.

Michelle remarked on the importance of a support network and relationships as she ages with HIV. She shared that her social support comes from the other women in her drug treatment program's group home and her doctor instead of from her family: "Now, my people will—not all the time—but like maybe once a year or so, they'll say, 'How your numbers doing, or how's your health?' Something like that, they'll ask, but as far as going to appointments and things or talking about the emotional part—but I also, early on, I thought it's too much to burden some of the other people."

Moreover, Michelle expressed her desire for a committed relationship to supplement her support network:

> I don't have a partner, and I really want a committed relationship. I just haven't found one yet. I want an older guy 'cause I'm an older woman. I'm 62, so I don't want anybody under 59. I hope God sends me a companion. I really do. I don't want a die alone, and I want to share with a man; a man and woman relationship is what I'm looking for. I don't want just a buddy pal. I want a strong, intimate relationship of somebody who understands and is concerned when I feel bad or anything like that. I want somebody that understands and still wants to spend time with me, even though I'm living with HIV.

The needs expressed by my interview participants to find supportive and knowledgeable healthcare and support services as they age with HIV were also identified as national needs. The next chapter summarizes key research findings and identifies areas where more research is needed to support the increasing number of people aging with HIV.

Chapter 12

Aging with HIV Research

As discussed further in this book's conclusion, one goal of the United States is to improve the health outcomes for positive people (The White House, 2021). To achieve this goal, as it relates to older people living with HIV, healthcare providers need to improve their HIV awareness and their ability to provide comprehensive care (The White House, 2021). This chapter focuses on some of the research in support of this goal of improving the health outcomes of people over 50 who are living with HIV. In this chapter, I examine some of the available research on the top three concerns of women aging with HIV: comorbidities, stigma, and the need for supportive services.

COMORBIDITIES

As people living with HIV age, they are more likely to suffer comorbidities that complicate their health and their treatment of HIV. Women living with HIV are especially susceptible to comorbidities, such as diabetes, high blood pressure, and stroke (The Well Project, 2022). For instance, the risk of a heart attack for postmenopausal, positive women is higher than for negative women because of a buildup of plaque in their blood vessels caused by the increased inflammation from HIV and because there are often no symptoms of heart problems before a heart attack (The Well Project, 2022).

Another comorbidity that affects postmenopausal women living with HIV is the formation of cancers, especially cervical, breast, colon, and anal (The Well Project, 2022). Older women living with HIV are also at higher risk of weakened bones and a loss of bone density, which leads to osteoporosis and possible fractures (The Well Project, 2022). Additionally, some women living with HIV suffer anemia, which may cause difficulty in thinking, a weakening of muscle strength, and an increased risk of falling (The Well Project, 2022).

Furthermore, postmenopausal women are especially vulnerable to becoming infected or reinfected with HIV and other sexually transmitted infections because they may not feel a need to use condoms during vaginal intercourse since they are not concerned about pregnancy after menopause (NIH, 2021). Also, as women age, their vaginas become thinner and drier, which can cause a tear during intercourse leading to a potential HIV transmission (NIH, 2021). Additionally, healthcare providers may not test older women for HIV, thinking they are at low risk of getting HIV and being hesitant to ask women about their sexual behaviors (NIH, 2021). Healthcare providers may also confuse the symptoms of HIV with the symptoms of aging, postponing the testing for HIV until it is at an advanced stage (NIH, 2021).

The effects of aging with HIV and the effects of comorbidities are still being investigated. Moreover, scientists are still determining the effects of HIV on the immune system and whether HIV causes a person to experience accelerated aging. According to The Well Project (2022), HIV activates the immune system, which results in an increased amount of inflammation throughout the body over an extended amount of time. This increased inflammation may lead to heart disease, cancer, and premature aging (The Well Project, 2022). Scientists still do not know the persistent effects of the antiretroviral medications people take to control HIV (The Well Project, 2022). Furthermore, the effects of the long-term use of antiretroviral therapies are especially under-researched in women, according to The Well Project (2022). In addition to the need to research the lasting effects of antiretroviral medications and the interaction of comorbidities and HIV, there is also a need for more research on the experience of ageism and HIV stigma, especially as sustained by women.

STIGMA

As people age in the United States, they often suffer ageism, encountering discrimination because their older age is viewed with negativity. Moreover, aging adults often lose their social networks and the support of family and friends. This loss of social networks may cause older people to isolate themselves from others, to feel ashamed, and to experience depression (The Well Project, 2022). Additionally, older people living with HIV may confront the compounding effects of HIV stigma in addition to ageism. They may find it difficult to connect with people who can support them, such as a mental health counselor, a case manager, or other older people living with HIV (The Well Project, 2022). According to de Mendonça Lima et al. (2021), one of the risk factors for suicide in older people is the experience of stigma, which exacerbates the social isolation and the lack of social integration already sustained as a person ages. Furthermore, because of intersectional stigma, the discrimination and marginalization already endured by people of color and LGBTQ+ people are compounded as they age (McCabe & Kinney, 2019).

Reducing the HIV-related stigma and discrimination suffered by positive people is another goal of the *National HIV/AIDS Strategy for the United States 2022–2025* (The White House, 2021). A key method to achieve this goal is to support communities that are most vulnerable to experiencing the compounding effects of intersectional stigma, especially people of color and people who are substance users (The White House, 2021). Another strategy is to educate and train healthcare professionals about HIV stigma, ageism, and the effects of marginalization, so they can better care for people aging with HIV who may be experiencing stigma (The White House, 2021). This social support is key to mitigating the effects of aging with HIV.

SUPPORTIVE SERVICES

There is a desperate need for more supportive services as people age in the United States. Furthermore, an increase in supportive social services will help to address the above concerns of comorbidities and stigma. According to de Mendonça Lima et al. (2021), older adults are more likely to ask and trust their primary care provider for medical advice because they have built a long-term relationship with them. For this reason, it is important that primary care providers receive ongoing training in both geriatrics and HIV to maximize their care and support (de Mendonça Lima et al., 2021). Moreover, primary care providers need additional training to recognize the effects of isolation, depression, and other potential mental health conditions, so they can address these concerns quickly and connect patients with specialists who can help them (de Mendonça Lima et al., 2021).

Improvements are also needed in the efforts to reduce isolation and to increase social support for aging adults. According to de Mendonça Lima et al. (2021), marriage acts as a protective factor against suicide and provides social support, reducing isolation. However, many people living with HIV are not in supportive partnerships and live in social isolation. This is especially true of older LGBTQ+ adults (McCabe & Kinney, 2019). To reduce isolation, communities can offer activities, supportive spaces, and affordable housing to connect older adults to others. According to McCabe and Kinney (2019), there is a need to increase supportive services for older adults in the United States because there is a lack of housing and community spaces that are welcoming and supportive of LGBTQ+ and older adults living with HIV. Additionally, as mentioned in the previous section, many LGBTQ+ and older adults living with HIV face stigma and discrimination while living in assisted care facilities and participating in community spaces.

The next chapter summarizes some research-based recommendations for individuals, communities, and society to implement as they develop the supportive services that will enhance the lives of women living with HIV.

Chapter 13

Developing HIV Endurance

As the number of older women living with HIV continues to grow, society must begin to address their unique needs. As discussed in chapter 12, these needs include treating comorbidities, reducing the stigma associated with aging and HIV, and providing the necessary supportive services to ensure women living with HIV are cared for as they age. This chapter offers some recommendations for individuals, organizations, and societies to implement to foster HIV endurance and to help women who are living with HIV age with grace, fulfillment, and well-being.

RECOMMENDATIONS FOR INDIVIDUALS

As mentioned in chapter 11, the women I interviewed credited living with HIV as helping them to find and renew their purpose in life. They reconnected with family and repaired relationships. Some women became advocates for HIV prevention and volunteered to educate and to help others in their communities. For example, Esther mentioned how volunteering with her local AIDS Service Organization helped her to live with a renewed purpose during her retirement: "I'm here volunteering; I've been here almost two years. It was positive, and we worked together here and all that. My parents are deceased, and I think that this is something that they would want me to do and continue to do." My findings support previous research by Dalmida et al. (2012) who determined that being diagnosed with HIV caused women to reexamine their spiritual beliefs and their lives. Additionally, Dalmida et al. (2012) identified living with a purpose, having inner peace, and finding support as some of the benefits of spirituality.

According to Gilbert and Wright (2003), after women are diagnosed with HIV, they often reevaluate their lives, change their circumstances, and reconnect spiritually. Some women leave abusive relationships, restore relationships with estranged family and friends, volunteer, and maintain sobriety

(Gilbert & Wright, 2003). For example, Ava revealed how meeting other women who were living with HIV helped her to change her lifestyle and find her life purpose:

> During that time, I wasn't [speaking about HIV]. Then, I got off of the pity party and said I should be saying [something]. So, I met some wonderful women, back during those years, and they supported me; and I'd seen how happy they were and prosperous, and how they could go out and speak; and it was like an ah-ha moment, like I need to do this, so that nobody else feels the way I feel ever again. I did not want another woman to suffer in silence like I did, for as long as I did.

Women who are aging with HIV are also concerned about comorbidities. They may experience diabetes, heart disease, dementia, and chronic pain. According to de Mendonça Lima et al. (2021), older women may also experience anxiety, depression, and isolation. To address these comorbidities, women who are aging with HIV need to receive regular medical care through their primary care physician and specialists who are knowledgeable about HIV and geriatrics. Women also need supportive relationships in their lives to keep them from living in social isolation. D'Amore (2019) recommends women living with HIV participate in support groups where they can speak with other women who are living with HIV. Support groups provide a place where women can learn positive coping strategies and share their lived experiences of aging and HIV. Women can attend support groups via social media or in person.

The next section suggests organizational and societal changes to address the needs of older women living with HIV.

RECOMMENDATIONS FOR ORGANIZATIONS AND SOCIETY

Because women who are aging with HIV encounter comorbidities, they need primary care providers and specialists who understand both geriatrics and HIV. Cahill and Krivo-Kaufman (2009) recommend increasing the number of geriatrics programs in medical schools and propose increasing the amount of information and training primary care providers and other healthcare practitioners receive regarding HIV and geriatrics care. This training would help to reduce the stigma associated with HIV and ageism while increasing the well-being of women by providing them with better healthcare.

To help women access knowledgeable healthcare providers who can treat their HIV and aging concerns, Aitcheson et al. (2014) recommend Medicaid be expanded through the Patient Protection and Affordable Care Act (2010) because positive people are three times more likely to rely on Medicaid than the general population. They also suggest increasing funding for the Ryan White programs, which provide support services and medical care that is especially important to people too young to enroll in Medicare (Aitcheson et al., 2014). Through the Ryan White AIDS Drug Assistance Program, older women living with HIV can get help paying for their antiretroviral medications, case management, and transportation assistance (Aitcheson et al., 2014).

Moreover, there is a great need for supportive housing and long-term care facilities that welcome people who are LGBTQ+, people of color, and people who are living with HIV (McCabe & Kinney, 2019). Because older people are more prone to social isolation and loneliness, they need facilities that are welcoming, affordable, free of discrimination, and operated by caring and knowledgeable personnel (de Mendonça Lima et al., 2021).

There is also a need to increase research on the effects of aging with HIV. Cahill and Krivo-Kaufman (2009) propose increasing the amount of clinical research targeted at positive people over the age of 50. Aitcheson et al. (2014) concur and suggest priority areas of research include the management of comorbidities, behavioral health needs, and caregiver support resources. This research especially needs to include marginalized and less studied groups, such as women of color and people who are LGBTQ+ (Aitcheson et al., 2014).

It is critical for individuals, organizations, and society to construct and employ structures to sustain HIV endurance, especially as more people are living longer with HIV. In summary, table 13.1 offers some additional suggestions for individuals, organizations, and society to help people living with HIV live longer and more fulfilling lives.

Table 13.1. Building and Sustaining HIV Endurance

Individuals	*Organizations*	*Society*
Find your purpose.	Welcome all people.	Eliminate laws that criminalize HIV transmission.
Join a support group.	Eliminate discrimination and stigma.	Focus more resources to develop improved antiretroviral medications and a vaccine for HIV.
Volunteer and serve others.	Provide workshops and trainings to educate people about HIV.	Provide supportive and affordable housing for people living and aging with HIV.
Take your medications faithfully.	Provide a living wage to employees.	Expand Medicaid and Medicare for people living and aging with HIV.
Employ your spiritual practices.	Provide health insurance and sick leave.	Ensure all eligible people living with HIV can receive and afford antiretroviral medications.
Educate yourself and others.	Be supportive and welcome diversity.	Increase the use of harm reduction practices when addressing the use of illegal drugs.

Personal Connection

Maintaining Social Capital

As our society begins to address the diversity of needs of the growing aging community, it is important to establish social institutions that can respond to the needs of people aging with HIV. It is critical to build community networks that connect vital social anchors and help to develop and maintain social capital. Clopton and Finch (2011) identified two main criteria for developing and maintaining social capital in institutions: (1) the need to establish trust and reciprocity, while embracing diversity across social networks, and (2) for social anchors in a community to create, enhance, and sustain a collective identity for individuals and the community.

Maintaining social capital requires individuals to connect with each other, and communities can help this process by providing social anchors where diverse individuals can meet. The Office of the U.S. Surgeon General (2023, p. 7) describes social capital as encompassing "both social support and social cohesion" and suggests that communities need to promote the "programs, policies, and physical elements" to provide the critical resources to enhance social capital. I am fortunate to live in a community that offers several social anchors and community places for me to use, which helps me to maintain my social capital as I age. For instance, I joined my local YMCA several years ago because I realized I needed more social interaction. Going to the YMCA connects me to other members of my community and allows me to engage in conversation with people who I normally would not speak to. Also, I have renewed my strength training efforts, which I had neglected for many years.

Another example of developing and maintaining my social capital is my use of the public library. I have always used several libraries in my area because they are great social anchors that are open community places where everyone is welcome. Public libraries offer books, audiobooks, meeting spaces, and computers, and I use their services several times each month. I have also enjoyed going to lectures, concerts, and movies at my community libraries.

Two other community organizations that help me to maintain my social capital are schools and churches. At both places, I encounter people who have different viewpoints and life experiences, but we are meeting for a similar purpose and in a common place. Listening to and speaking with other people helps me to see beyond our differences and establish relationships.

Some other activities that help me develop and maintain my social capital are visiting with my family and friends and enjoying meals together. I also enjoy walking around my neighborhood and speaking with my neighbors. Occasionally, I help to distribute food at a food bank. I also try to attend community festivals and concerts where I can interact with other people who live in my community.

The Office of the U.S. Surgeon General (2023, p. 47) identified "six pillars to advance social connection." The examples I gave above of my efforts to sustain social capital connect to the first pillar, which is to strengthen social infrastructure in local communities (Office of the U.S. Surgeon General, 2023, p. 47). As organizations and communities enhance their community spaces and build their social infrastructure to meet the needs of an aging population, they will encourage more people to connect with each other. It is important for these community spaces to be safe, accessible, and welcoming to all, especially people who are aging, people living with HIV, and people who identify as LGBTQ+. As more organizations and communities create opportunities for people to connect with and know each other better, social capital will increase. This social capital is important to help reduce the isolation caused by aging.

Four Key Takeaways

HIV and Aging

- As a woman ages with HIV, she needs healthcare providers and other supportive services that can address the overlapping concerns of HIV, geriatrics, and comorbidities.
- Some women aging with HIV find purpose in their lives through family relationships, volunteering, participating in support groups, and educating others about HIV prevention.
- Organizations and society can help people who are aging with HIV by creating welcoming and supportive community spaces free of ageism and HIV stigma.
- As women age with HIV, they need supportive and affordable housing and long-term care facilities that are free from discrimination, along with affordable prescriptions and financial stability.

Conclusion

The four sections of this book focused on the experiences of women living with HIV in the areas of disclosing HIV, managing HIV stigma, incorporating HIV into identity, and aging with HIV. These areas of focus are similar to the four goals proposed by the *National HIV/AIDS Strategy for the United States 2022–2025* [*Strategy*]. The four goals are: "(1) prevent new HIV infections, (2) improve HIV-related health outcomes of people with HIV, (3) reduce HIV-related disparities and health inequities, and (4) achieve integrated, coordinated efforts that address the HIV epidemic among all partners and interested parties" (The White House, 2021, pp. 3–10). These four goals and their subgoals attempt to outline the steps needed to achieve the *Strategy's* vision statement, which is: "The United States will be a place where new HIV infections are prevented, every person knows their status, and every person with HIV has high-quality care and treatment, lives free from stigma and discrimination, and can achieve their full potential for health and well-being across the lifespan." (The White House, 2021, p. 1). The *Strategy* goes onto declare: "This vision includes all people, regardless of age, sex, gender identity, sexual orientation, race, ethnicity, religion, disability, geographic location, or socioeconomic circumstance." (The White House, 2021, p. 1).

In addition, one of the key indicators the *Strategy* lists to identify progress towards these four goals is to "decrease stigma among people with diagnosed HIV by 50% from a 2018 baseline median score of 31.2 on a 10-item questionnaire" (The White House, 2021, p. 11). To reduce stigma, the *Strategy* advocates for the removal of state laws and policies that criminalize behavior that may or may not lead to HIV transmission (The White House, 2021). Two other recommendations are to strengthen civil rights laws to protect positive people and to increase training for healthcare professionals to improve their understanding of the effects of HIV stigma and discrimination (The White House, 2021). The *Strategy* also emphasizes the need to provide more funding and resources to marginalized communities to help address and mitigate the HIV stigma these groups face (The White House, 2021).

One of the key objectives for the second goal of improving the "HIV-related health outcomes of people with HIV" (The White House, 2021, p. 39) is to "expand capacity to provide whole-person care to older adults with HIV and long-term survivors" (The White House, 2021, p. 39). To address this objective, the *Strategy* encourages more training for people who service and support positive people, especially in areas where there is a shortage of knowledgeable healthcare providers (The White House, 2021). This training can help educate providers about the unique needs of people aging with HIV. Through increased training, healthcare providers can learn how to better treat positive women who are living with comorbidities, such as diabetes, cancer, heart disease, and dementia. In addition, case managers and other supportive services can create systems to help women manage multiple prescriptions and to reduce the social isolation marginalized communities experience (The White House, 2021).

To achieve comprehensive care, support services also need to address the needs of some people living with HIV, such as transportation, affordable housing, mental health, and nutrition (The White House, 2021). Furthermore, women living with HIV need to create and contribute to more support groups for women living with HIV, where they can speak to other women about living and aging with HIV (D'Amore, 2019). These groups help women become more comfortable disclosing their HIV status, managing HIV stigma, incorporating HIV into their identities, and aging with HIV. In addition, support groups empower women to speak publicly about HIV prevention and provide them a space to network with and educate others, which empowers women and helps them to build HIV endurance (D'Amore, 2019).

Appendix A

List of Resources

AIDS Law Project of Pennsylvania
1211 Chestnut St., Suite 600
Philadelphia, PA 19107
215-587-9377
www.aidslawpa.org
Advocating for legal rights

AVAC: Global Advocacy for HIV Prevention
423 West 127th St., 4th Fl.
New York, NY 10027
212-796-6423
www.avac.org
Advocating for HIV treatment

Black AIDS Institute (BAI)
3894 Crenshaw Blvd., #56858
Los Angeles, CA 90056
info@BlackAIDS.org
blackaids.org
Focused on ending HIV in Black communities

HIV Nightline Crisis Line
1-800-628-9240
415-434-2437
Responds to calls 24/7

National Association of People with AIDS (NAPWA)
8401 Colesville Rd., Suite 505
Silver Spring, MD 20910
1-866-846-9366; 240-247-0574
www.napwa.org
Empowers individuals through information

National Black Leadership Commission on Health, Inc. (Black Health, Inc.)
215 West 125th St., 2nd Fl.
New York, NY 10027
212-614-0023
info@nblch.org
nblch.org
Focused on health equity

National Coalition of 100 Black Women, Inc. (NCBW)
1720 Peachtree Street NW, Suite 1020
Atlanta, GA 30309
404-390-3982
ncbw.org
Promotes leadership development

Positive Women's Network—USA
436 14th St., Suite 425
Oakland, CA 94612
info@pwn-usa.org
www.pwn-usa.org
Empowering positive women

POZ
Smart + Strong
157 Columbus Ave., Suite 525
New York, NY 10023–6082
212-242-2163
www.poz.com
Provides HIV information

Rural Women's Health Project
1108 SW Second Ave.
Gainesville, FL 32601
352-372-1095
info@rwhp.org
www.rwhp.org
Focused on health justice for immigrants

SAGE: Advocacy & Services for LGBTQ+ Elders
305 Seventh Ave., 15th Fl.
New York, NY 10001
1-877-360-LGBT(5428)
212-741-2247
www.sageusa.org
Advocating for LGBTQ+ rights

SisterLove, Inc.
PO Box 10558
1237 Ralph David Abernathy Blvd., SW
Atlanta, GA 30310
1-866-750-7733
404-505-7777
www.sisterlove.org
Advocating for women's health

The Body: The HIV/AIDS Resource
461 Fifth Ave., 14th Fl.
New York, NY 10017
212-695-2223
www.thebody.com
Provides HIV education to the public

The Graying of AIDS
info@grayingofaids.org
www.grayingofaids.org
Provides resources for adults over age 50

WORLD
389 30th St.
Oakland, CA 94609
510-986-0340
womenhiv.org
Focus on improving women's health

Appendix B

Relevant HIV-Related Terms

(Source: Office of AIDS Research. (2021). *Glossary of HIV/AIDS-Related Terms 2021* (9th ed.). National Institutes of Health. clinicalinfo.hiv.gov/en/glossary)

Acquired Immunodeficiency Syndrome (AIDS) = AIDS is the most advanced stage of HIV infection where a person's CD4 count is less than 200 cells/mm3 or the person has an AIDS-defining condition, such as opportunistic infections, cancers, or life-threatening conditions.
AIDS Service Organization (ASO) = AIDS Service Organizations are non-governmental organizations that provide services connected to the prevention and treatment of HIV/AIDS.
Antiretroviral Therapy = An antiretroviral drug is used to prevent a retrovirus like HIV from replicating. Antiretroviral therapy is also known as combination therapy or highly active antiretroviral therapy because a person usually takes three antiretroviral drugs from at least two different HIV drug groups.
Centers for Disease Control and Prevention (CDC) = This federal agency protects the health and safety of people by disseminating information to prevent and control diseases.
Comorbidity = A comorbid condition is when a person has two or more diseases or conditions at the same time.
Condom = A prophylactic that may prevent the transmission of sexually transmitted infections, such as HIV, when used during vaginal, anal, or oral sex.
Drug Class = Antiretroviral drugs to treat HIV are divided into seven drug classes based on how each drug interferes with HIV's life cycle. The seven classes are: nucleoside reverse transcriptase inhibitors (NRTIs), non-nucleoside reverse transcriptase inhibitors (NNRTIs), protease inhibitors (PIs), fusion inhibitors, CCR5 antagonists, post-attachment inhibitors, and integrase strand transfer inhibitors (INSTIs).

Genital Warts = A sexually transmitted infection caused by the human papillomavirus (HPV), which causes raised flesh-colored bumps on the surface of the tissue surrounding the vagina, cervix, tip of the penis, or anus.
Human Immunodeficiency Virus (HIV) = HIV is a retrovirus that occurs as two types: HIV-1, which is most common in the United States, and HIV-2, which is most common in West Africa. Both types are transmitted through direct contact with body fluids containing HIV. These body fluids include blood, semen, vaginal fluids, and breast milk.
Pap Test = This procedure, also known as a Pap smear, collects cells and secretions from inside and around the cervix to determine if there are any precancerous or cancerous cells
Pneumonia = Bronchopneumonia inflammation of the lungs is caused by a bacterial, viral, or fungal infection, and if a person with HIV gets recurrent pneumonia, it is considered an AIDS-defining condition. Symptoms of pneumonia include coughing, shortness of breath, fevers, chills, chest pain, and weakness.
Post-Exposure Prophylaxis (PEP) = A short-term treatment that is started as soon as possible after a high-risk exposure to HIV or other infectious agents, such as hepatitis B or C viruses. The purpose of this treatment is to reduce the risk of infection.
Pre-Exposure Prophylaxis (PrEP) = A prevention method for people who are HIV negative and who are at high risk of getting infected with HIV. PrEP involves taking a specific combination of HIV medications each day.
President's Emergency Plan for AIDS Relief (PEPFAR) = A global initiative to combat the HIV/AIDS epidemic by working with governmental and non-governmental partners to support HIV prevention, treatment, and care programs around the world, with a focus on women, children, and men who have sex with men.
Rapid Test = A rapid HIV antibody test can detect HIV antibodies in blood or oral fluid in less than 30 minutes.
Ryan White HIV/AIDS Program = The largest federally funded program that provides HIV-related services to low-income, uninsured, and underinsured people who are living with HIV. The program is also known as the Care Act, and its services are available in all 50 states, US territories, and the District of Columbia.
Stigma = Stigma refers to the negative beliefs and assumptions people associate with a specific situation, characteristic, condition, or person. Experiencing HIV stigma can result in negative health effects, affecting the well-being of a person living with HIV.

T Lymphocyte (T Cell) = There are two types of T lymphocytes: CD8 cells and CD4 cells. HIV infects and destroys CD4 cells, which gradually destroys the immune system.

Undetectable Viral Load = A person's viral load is considered undetectable when the amount of HIV in the blood is too low to be detected with a viral load (HIV RNA) test. A person's viral load is reported as the number of HIV RNA copies per milliliter of blood. A viral load test is used to diagnose an HIV infection and monitor the response to antiretroviral therapy. By maintaining an undetectable viral load, a person living with HIV is unable to sexually transmit the virus, which is known as Undetectable = Untransmittable (U = U).

Appendix C

Spiritual Principles and Attitudinal Pillars of Mindfulness

(Source: Dunnavent, L. B. (2003). *Spiritual Development* [presentation]. Spiritual Development Workshops, Harrisburg, PA, United States.)

Be Here Now (Pillar: Beginner's Mind)	*Being in the Now gives us a vast amount of time.* • Value and enjoy each moment. • See everything as if it were your first time. • Be a good listener and give your undivided attention.
Kindness Towards Self, Loved Ones, Neutral People, and Enemies (Pillar: Nonjudging)	*May ______ be happy. May ______ be free of suffering. May ______ be at peace.* • Love yourself and love your neighbor as yourself. • Forgive yourself and others. • Observe the judgments you make.
Developing the Attitude of Gratitude (Pillar: Be Thankful)	*Do as much as you can, in the time you have, in the place you are.* • Appreciate each moment and person in your life. • There is a light inside all of us. • The worst experiences and people are our best teachers in life.
Developing Patience (Pillar: Patience and Tolerance)	*We are dependent on each other for everything. We are responsible for each other.* • Patience is an attitude and a form of wisdom. • Practice wait time. • Before you speak, ask yourself if what you are about to say is a lie, divisive, offensive, or senseless? • Experience is determined by you, not your life circumstances.
Acceptance of Self, Others, and What Is (Pillar: Acceptance and Non-Striving)	*Acceptance brings peacefulness and calmness.* • Be open and see things as they are. • You are human and divine. • Everyone's life is equally hard.

Developing Compassion (Pillar: Nonjudging)	*Help other people and relieve their pain through your service to others.* • Compassion is feeling empathy for others. • Care about another person because it could be you. • Whether good or bad comes out of darkness depends on us and what we do. • Have a deep respect for ourselves and others.
Developing the Attitude of Forgiveness (Pillar: Letting Go)	*Forgiveness is unconditional love.* • Forgiveness provides closure. If you don't forgive, you are chained to the person or action. • Each person has their own attachments. • Let go and live in the present. • Let go of old attachments, patterns, and beliefs to step into freedom and grace.
Developing the Attitude of Love (Pillar: Trust)	*Love unconditionally.* • Love now is real. • Cultivate a trusting heart, and trust and believe in yourself. • The more you fear, the less you trust. • Humble yourself and open your heart. • Love is the hardest lesson.

References

Allen, M., Emmers-Sommer, T. M., Sahlstein, E., & Valde, K. (2012). Managing boundaries of a life with HIV. In K. L. Walker, J. L. Hart, & M. U. D'Silva (Eds.), *Communicating about HIV/AIDS: Taboo topics and forbidden conversations* (pp. 79–93). Hampton Press.

Altman, I., & Taylor, D. A. (1973). *Social penetration: The development of interpersonal relationships*. Holt, Rinehart & Winston.

Americans With Disabilities Act of 1990, Pub. L. No. 101–336, 104 Stat. 328. (1990). https://www.ada.gov/pubs/adastatute08.htm

amfAR. (2022, June). *Snapshots of an Epidemic: An HIV/AIDS Timeline*. Snapshots of an Epidemic: An HIV/AIDS Timeline—amfAR, The Foundation for AIDS Research. https://www.amfar.org/about-hiv-aids/hiv-aids-snapshots-of-an-epidemic/

Aitcheson, P., Brennan-Ing, M., Espinoza, R., Pacheco, B, Tax, A., & Tietz, D. (2014). *Eight policy recommendations for improving the health and wellness of older adults with HIV*. Diverse Elders Coalition. https://diverseelders.org/

Berger, M. T. (2004). *Workable sisterhood: The political journey of stigmatized women with HIV/AIDS*. Princeton University Press.

Borger, I. (Ed.). (1996). *From a burning house: The AIDS Project Los Angeles Workshop collection*. Washington Square Press.

Boss, P. (2007). Ambiguous loss theory: Challenges for scholars and practitioners. *Family Relations, 56*(2), 105–111. https://doi.org/10.1111/j.1741-3729.2007.00444.x

Bray, P. (2010). A broader framework for exploring the influence of spiritual experience in the wake of stressful life events: Examining connections between post-traumatic growth and psycho-spiritual transformation. *Mental Health, Religion & Culture, 13*(3), 293–308. https://doi.org/10.1080/13674670903367199

Bury, M. (1982). Chronic illness as biographical disruption. *Sociology of Health and Illness, 4*, 167–82. https://doi.org/10.1111/1467-9566.ep11339939

Bury, M. (1991). The sociology of chronic illness: A review of research and prospects. *Sociology of Health & Illness, 13*(4), 451–68. https://doi.org/10.1111/j.1467-9566.1991.tb00522.x

Cahill, S. & Krivo-Kaufman, A. (2009). Growing older with HIV. *Achieve*, 1–4. AIDS Community Research Initiative of America and Gay Men's Health Crisis.

Centers for Disease Control and Prevention. (2022a). *HIV and women.* https://www.cdc.gov/hiv/group/gender/women/incidence.html
Centers for Disease Control and Prevention. (2022b). *HIV by age: HIV diagnoses.* https://www.cdc.gov/hiv/group/age/diagnoses.html
Charmaz, K. (1983). Loss of self: A fundamental form of suffering in the chronically ill. *Sociology of Health and Illness, 5*(2), 168–95. https://doi.org/10.1111/1467-9566.ep10491512
Charmaz, K. (1991). *Good days, bad days: The self in chronic illness and time.* Rutgers University Press.
Charmaz, K. (1994). Identity dilemmas of chronically ill men. *The Sociological Quarterly, 35*(2), 269–88. https://doi.org/10.1111/j.1533-8525.1994.tb00410.x
Charmaz, K. (2002). The self as habit: The reconstruction of self in chronic illness. *OTJR: Occupation, Participation, and Health, 22*(1_suppl), 31S–41S. https://doi.org/10.1177/15394492020220s105
Charmaz, K. (2008). Views from the margins: Voices, silences, and suffering. *Qualitative Research in Psychology, 5*, 7–18. https://doi.org/10.1080/14780880701863518
Charmaz, K. (2009). Stories and silences: Disclosures and self in chronic illness. In D. E. Brashers, & D. J. Goldsmith (Eds.), *Communicating to manage health and illness* (pp. 240–70). Routledge.
Chaudoir, S. R., & Fisher, J. D. (2010). The disclosure processes model: Understanding disclosure decision-making and post-disclosure outcomes among people living with a concealable stigmatized identity. *Psychological Bulletin, 136*(2), 236–56. https://doi.org/10.1037/a0018193
Chaudoir, S. R., Fisher, J. D., & Simoni, J. M. (2011). Understanding HIV disclosure: A review and application of the disclosure processes model. *Social Science and Medicine, 72*(10), 1618–29. https://doi.org/10.1016/j.socscimed.2011.03.028
Ciambrone, D. (2003). *Women's experiences with HIV/AIDS: Mending fractured selves.* Haworth Press.
Clopton, A. W. & Finch, B. L. (2011). Re-conceptualizing social anchors in community development: Utilizing social anchor theory to create social capital's third dimension. *Community Development: Journal of the Community Development Society, 42*(1), 70–83. https://doi.org/10.1080/15575330.2010.505293
Collins, P. H. (1990). Black feminist epistemology. In C. Calhoun, J. Gerteis, J. Moody, S. Pfaff, & I. Virk (Eds.), *Contemporary sociological theory* (3rd ed., pp. 407–16). Wiley-Blackwell.
Crenshaw, K. W. (1994). Mapping the margins: Intersectionality, identity politics, and violence against women of color. In M. A. Fineman & R. Mykitiuk (Eds.), *The public nature of private violence* (pp. 93–118). Routledge.
Crockett, P. H. (1997). *HIV law: A survival guide to the legal system for people living with HIV.* Three Rivers Press.
D'Amore, C.F. (2019). *Unmasking HIV: Women and experiences of disclosure* (Publication No. 22584161) [Doctoral dissertation, Indiana University of Pennsylvania]. ProQuest.

D'Amore, C. F. (2021). Mindful leadership: Transform your self, organization, and society. In T. Mengel (Ed.), *Leadership for the future: Lessons from the past, current approaches, and future insights*. (pp. 87–110). Cambridge Scholars.

Dalmida, S. G., Holstad, M. M., Dilorio, C., & Laderman, G. (2012). The meaning and use of spirituality among African American women living with HIV/AIDS. *Western Journal of Nursing Research, 34*(6), 736–65. https://doi.org/10.1177/0193945912443740

de Mendonça Lima, C. A., De Leo, D., Ivbijaro, G., & Svab, I. (2021). Suicide prevention in older adults. *Asia Pacific Psychiatry, 13*(3), e12473. https://doi.org/10.1111/appy.12473

Derlega, V. J., Winstead, B. A., Greene, K., Serovich, J., & Elwood, W. N. (2004). Reasons for HIV disclosure/nondisclosure in close relationships: Testing a model of HIV-disclosure decision making. *Journal of Social and Clinical Psychology, 23*(6), 747–77. https://doi.org/10.1521/jscp.23.6.747.54804

Dunnavent, L. B. (2003). *Spiritual Development* [presentation]. Spiritual Development Workshops, Harrisburg, PA.

Farmer, P., Connors, M., & Simmons, J. (Eds.). (2011). *Women, poverty, and AIDS: Sex, drugs, and structural violence* (2nd ed.). Common Courage Press.

Feldman, D. A., & Miller, J. W. (Eds.). (1998). *The AIDS crisis: A documentary history*. Greenwood Press.

Fesko, S. L. (2001). Disclosure of HIV status in the workplace: Considerations and strategies. *Health & Social Work, 26*(4), 235–44. https://doi.org/10.1093/hsw/26.4.235

Foster, P. P., & Gaskins, S. W. (2009). Older African Americans' management of HIV/AIDS stigma. *AIDS Care, 21*(10), 1306–12. https://doi.org/10.1080/09540120902803141

Frank, A. W. (1995). *The wounded storyteller: Body, illness, and ethics*. University of Chicago Press.

Gilbert, D. J., & Wright, E. M. (Eds.). (2003). *African American women and HIV/AIDS: Critical responses*. Praeger Press.

Goffman, E. (1959). *The presentation of self in everyday life*. Doubleday Anchor Books.

Goffman, E. (1963). *Stigma: Notes on the management of spoiled identity*. Prentice-Hall.

Greene, K., Magsamen-Conrad, K., Venetis, M. K., Checton, M. G., Bagdasarov, Z., & Banerjee, S. C. (2012). Accessing health diagnosis disclosure decisions in relationships: Testing the disclosure decision-making model. *Health Communication, 27*, 356–68. https://doi.org/10.1080/10410236.2011.586988

Grof, S., & Grof, C. (1990). *The stormy search for self: A guide to personal growth through transformational crises*. JP Tarcher.

Habermas, J. (1996). Civil society and the political public sphere. In C. Calhoun, J. Gerteis, J. Moody, S. Pfaff, & I. Virk (Eds.), *Contemporary sociological theory* (3rd ed., pp. 469–89). Wiley-Blackwell.

Herek, G. M. (1999). AIDS and stigma. *The American Behavioral Scientist, 42*(7), 1106–16. https://doi.org/10.1177/0002764299042007004

Herron, L., Mutch, A., Mugamu, M., Howard, C., & Fitzgerald, L. (2022). The spiral just keeps on going: Cascading health and social issues for women living and aging with HIV. *Women's Health, 18,* 1–12. https://doi.org/10.1177/17455065221074882

HIV.gov. (2020, February 24). *Standing up to stigma*. https://www.hiv.gov/hiv-basics/overview/making-a-difference/standing-up-to-stigma

Kidd, R., & Clay, S. (2003, September). *Understanding and challenging HIV stigma: Toolkit for action. Trainers' guide*. Washington, D.C.: ICRW, The CHANGE Project. http://www.changeproject.org

Lau-Ng, R., Day, H., & Alford, D. P. (2020). Barriers facing older adults with substance use disorders in post-acute care settings. *Generations Journal of the American Society on Aging, 44*(4), 1–10. www.generations.asaging.org

Lazzarini, Z., Galletly, C. L., Mykhalovskiy, E., Harsono, D., O'Keefe, E., Singer, M., & Levine, R. J. (2013). Criminalization of HIV transmission and exposure: Research and policy agenda. *American Journal of Public Health, 103*(8), 1350–53. https://doi.org/10.2105/ajph.2013.301267

Lehman, J. S., Carr, M. H., Nichol, A. J., Ruisanchez, A., Knight, D. W., Langford, A. E., Gray, S. C., & Mermin, J. H. (2014). Prevalence and public health implications of state laws that criminalize potential HIV exposure in the United States. *AIDS and Behavior, 18*(6), 997–1006. https://doi.org/10.1007/s10461-014-0724-0

McCabe, H. A., & Kinney, M. K. (2019). LGBTQ+ individuals, health inequities, and policy implications. *Creighton Law Review, 52*, 427–50.

Moskowitz, D. A., & Roloff, M. E. (2012). On the HIV serodiscordant romantic relationship. In K. L. Walker, J. L. Hart, & M. U. D'Silva, M. U. (Eds.), *Communicating about HIV/AIDS: Taboo topics and forbidden conversations* (pp. 61–78). Hampton Press.

National Institutes of Health. (2021). *HIV and older people*. https://hivinfo.nih.gov/understanding-hiv/fact-sheets/hiv-and-older-people

Nixon, S., & Renwick, R. (2003). Experiences of contemplating returning to work for people living with HIV/AIDS. *Qualitative Health Research, 13*(9), 1272–90. https://doi.org/10.1177/1049732303257190

Nyblade, L., & MacQuarrie, K. (2006, January). *Can we measure HIV/AIDS-related stigma and discrimination? Current knowledge about qualifying stigma in developing countries*. Washington, D.C.: USAID, ICRW, POLICY Project. http://www.icrw.org/sites/default/files/publications/Can-We-Measure-HIV-Stigma-and-Discrimination.pdf

Office of the U.S. Surgeon General. (2023). *Our epidemic of loneliness and isolation: The U.S. Surgeon General's advisory on the healing effects of social connection and community*. Author. www.hhs.gov/surgeongeneral/priorities/connection/index.htm

Ogden, J., & Nyblade, L. (2005). *Common at its core: HIV-related stigma across contexts*. Washington, D.C.: International Center for Research on Women. http://www.icrw.org/sites/default/files/publications/Common-at-its-Core-HIV-Related-Stigma-Across-Contexts.pdf

Omarzu, J. (2000). A disclosure decision model: Determining how and when individuals will self-disclose. *Personality and Social Psychology Review, 4*(2), 174–85. https://doi.org/10.1207/s15327957pspr0402_05

Pargament, K. I. (1997). *The psychology of religion and coping: Theory, research, practice*. Guilford Press.

Patient Protection and Affordable Care Act of 2010, Pub. L. No. 111–148, 124 Stat. 119 (2010). https://www.congress.gov/111/plaws/publ148/PLAW-111publ148.pdf

Pellowski, J. A., Kalichman, S. C., Matthews, K. A., & Adler, N. (2013). A pandemic of the poor: Social disadvantage and the U.S. HIV epidemic. *American Psychologist, 68*(4), 197–209. https://doi.org/10.1037/a0032694

Persons, E., Kershaw, T., Sikkema, K. J., & Hansen, N. B. (2010). The impact of shame on health-related quality of life among HIV-positive adults with a history of childhood sexual abuse. *AIDS Patient Care and STDs, 24*(9), 571–80. https://doi.org/10.1089/apc.2009.0209

Qiao, S., Xiaoming, L., & Stanton, B. (2013). Theoretical models of parental HIV disclosure: A critical review. *AIDS Care, 25*(3), 326–36. https://doi.org/10.1080/09540121.2012.712658

Rendina, H. J., Weaver, L., Millar, B. M., Lopez-Matos, J., & Parsons, J. T. (2019). Psychosocial well-being and HIV-related immune health outcomes among HIV-positive older adults: Support for a biopsychological model of HIV stigma and health. *Journal of the International Association of Providers of AIDS Care, 18*, 1–11. https://doi.org/10.1177/2325958219888462

Rintamaki, L. S. (2009). The HIV social identity model. In D. E. Brashers, and D. J. Goldsmith (Eds.), *Communicating to manage health and illness* (pp. 212–39). Routledge.

Rintamaki, L. S., & Weaver, F. M. (2008). The social and personal dynamics of HIV stigma. In T. Edgar, S. M. Noar, & V. S. Freimuth (Eds.), *Communication perspectives on HIV/AIDS for the 21st century* (pp. 67–99). Taylor & Francis.

Romeyn, M. (1998). *Nutrition and HIV: A new model for treatment*. Jossey-Bass.

Sandelowski, M., Lambe, C., & Barroso, J. (2004). Stigma in HIV-positive women. *Journal of Nursing Scholarship, 36*(2), 122–28. https://doi.org/10.1111/j.1547-5069.2004.04024.x

Seidman, I. (2013). *Interviewing as qualitative research: A guide for researchers in education and the social sciences* (4th ed.). Teachers College Press.

Serovich, J. M., Craft, S. M., & Reed, S. J. (2012). Women's HIV disclosure to family and friends. *AIDS Patient Care and STDs, 26*(4), 241–49. doi: 10.1089/apc.2011.0319

Smith, R. A., Rossetto, K. R., & Peterson, B. L. (2012). HIV/AIDS, stigma, and communication. In K. L. Walker, J. L. Hart, & M. U. D'Silva (Eds.), *Communicating about HIV/AIDS: Taboo topics and forbidden conversations* (pp. 165–87). Hampton Press.

Spence, A. B., Wang, C., Michel, K., Ocampo, J. M., Kharfen, M., Merenstein, D., Goparaju, L., & Kassaye, S. (2022). HIV related stigma among healthcare providers: Opportunities for education and training. *Journal of the International Association of Providers of AIDS Care, 21*, 1–8. https://doi.org/10.1177/23259582221114797

Stets, J. E., & Burke, P. J. (2000). Identity theory and social identity theory. *Social Psychology Quarterly, 63*(3), 224–37. https://doi.org/10.2307/2695870

Tedeschi, R. G., & Calhoun, L. G. (1995). *Trauma & transformation: Growing in the aftermath of suffering*. SAGE.

Tedeschi, R. G., Park, C. L., & Calhoun, L. G. (1998). *Posttraumatic growth: Positive changes in the aftermath of crisis*. Lawrence Erlbaum Associates.

The Well Project. (2022). *Aging and HIV*. https://www.thewellproject.org/hiv-information/aging-and-hiv.

The White House. (2021). *National HIV/AIDS Strategy for the United States 2022–2025*. Washington, DC. https://www.whitehouse.gov/wp-content/uploads/2021/11/National-HIV-AIDS-Strategy.pdf

Timmons, J. C., & Fesko, S. L. (2004). The impact, meaning, and challenges of work: Perspectives of individuals with HIV/AIDS. *Health & Social Work, 29*(2), 137–44. https://doi.org/10.1093/hsw/29.2.137

Tsarenko, Y., & Polonsky, M. J. (2011). 'You can spend your life dying or you can spend your life living': Identity transition in people who are HIV-positive. *Psychology and Health, 26*(4), 465–83. https://doi.org/10.1080/08870440903521761

U.S. Department of Justice. (2008). *Americans with Disabilities Act of 1990, as amended in 2008*. https://www.ada.gov/law-and-regs/ada/

Vann-Ward, T., Morse, J. M., & Charmaz, K. (2017). Preserving self: Theorizing the social and psychological processes of living with Parkinson disease. *Qualitative Health Research, 27*(7), 964–82. https://doi.org/10.1177/1049732317707494

Index

About the Author

Living and aging with HIV since 1998, **Charlene F. D'Amore**, PhD speaks publicly about HIV prevention. Over the years, she has educated herself about HIV by attending conferences and through extensive reading. D'Amore earned her doctorate in 2019 with a dissertation focused on the disclosure experiences of women living with HIV. Her dissertation research is the basis for this book. Dr. D'Amore's research interests include the experience of HIV disclosure, HIV's effect on identity, HIV stigma, and the effects of aging with HIV. As a teacher in public education, Dr. D'Amore loves working with and teaching students in grades K to 12 and adults to read, write, and speak English. Dr. D'Amore has no conflicts of interest to disclose. You can contact Dr. D'Amore at HIVendurance@gmail.com. and connect with her on LinkedIn. She welcomes your feedback on this book.

www.ingramcontent.com/pod-product-compliance
Ingram Content Group UK Ltd.
Pitfield, Milton Keynes, MK11 3LW, UK
UKHW041839031026
15587UKWH00002B/884

9 781666 918618